Skills for Therapy Managers

The Essential Guide *to* Recruitment *and* Retention

Shelley Cohen, RN, BS, CEN • Dennis Sherrod, EdD, RN

with Nancy J. Beckley, MS, MBA, CHC

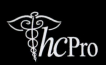

The Essential Guide to Recruitment and Retention: Skills for Therapy Managers is published
by HCPro, Inc.

ISBN 978-1-60146-102-5

HCPro, Inc., provides information resources for the healthcare industry.

HCPro, Inc., is not affiliated in any way with The Joint Commission, which owns the JCAHO
and Joint Commission trademarks.

Shelley Cohen, RN, BS, CEN, Co-author   Janell Lukac, Layout Artist
Dennis Sherrod, EdD, RN, Co-author   Audrey Doyle, Copyeditor
Nancy J. Beckley, MS, MBA, CHC, Co-author   Liza Banks, Proofreader
Patty Haggen, Reviewer   Darren Kelly, Books Production Supervisor
Adrienne Trivers, Editor   Susan Darbyshire, Art Director
Elizabeth Petersen, Executive Editor   Claire Cloutier, Production Manager
Emily Sheahan, Group Publisher   Jean St. Pierre, Director of Operations
Susan Darbyshire, Cover Designer

Advice given is general. Readers should consult professional counsel for specific legal, ethical,
or clinical questions.

Arrangements can be made for quantity discounts. For more information, contact:

HCPro, Inc.
P.O. Box 1168
Marblehead, MA 01945
Telephone: 800/650-6787 or 781/639-1872
Fax: 781/639-2982
E-mail: *customerservice@hcpro.com*

Visit HCPro at its World Wide Web sites:
www.hcpro.com and www.hcmarketplace.com

Table of contents

The Essential Guide to Recruitment and Retention

A word from the co-author

My first job as a therapist was in a hospital. By the next year I was the department head busy recruiting and hiring staff. This came at a time when I was trying to figure out the hospital's operating and capital budgeting process, how to requisition departmental supplies, the long-range planning process, new-employee orientation, how to implement progressive discipline, balance the chemicals in the therapy pool, as well as having to convince the risk management director that I needed to implement a pet therapy as well as wheelchair sports program.

It seems like I worked 12 hour days just trying to figure out everything, and just when I thought I might hit my rhythm the nation began experiencing a therapy shortage. I experienced the highs and lows of expensive advertising in the newspaper as well as the therapy publications, the trips to conventions with recruitment in mind, competing with recruitment and sign-on bonuses, continuing education packages, and moving packages (all of which my hospital didn't have).

Every day that a therapy position is open is another day when the rehab department scrambles to get all patient evaluations and therapy done while short-staffed, not to mention the pressure from finance on not meeting revenue projections. All this while administration is looking to you, the departmental manager, as the expert in keeping your department fully staffed and happy.

Studies have consistently shown that salary and compensation are further down the list of the top items that lead to job satisfaction. This is where the aspect of employee retention becomes paramount. It is so much better to tap into those elements that provide personal and professional job satisfaction. This book is an adaptation of HCPro's A Practical Guide to Recruitment and Retention: Skills for Nurse Managers written by Shelley Cohen and Dennis Sherrod.

The technology of today's workplace allows a vast array of recruiting sources, everything from video resumes on sites like YouTube to job and resume postings on sites like Monster. com. The aspect of retention still largely remains embedded in the personal and professional relationship that your staff has with you, the department, and the organization. Let this book help you get started with that process.

Nancy J. Beckley
September 2007

The revolving door

Make the change: You can stop the door from revolving

How many times have you promised yourself that next time you will handle things differently? Yet when that time approaches, it's easy to revert back to our old and comfortable behaviors.

Now is the time for you to commit to changing your recruitment and retention attitude and behavior. At a time when the facility down the street may simply dangle a recruitment bonus to recruit staff, you need ammunition you can dangle back to keep staff from moving out the door. Therefore, recruitment and retention needs your ongoing attention.

The disadvantages of high turnover

For every therapist you keep, consider the savings in time and money that did not have to go toward hiring and orienting a replacement therapist. Also, consider that lower turnover places less stress on the existing staff. As managers, we know all too well that staff members already feel overwhelmed by their daily responsibilities. For most of them, covering the patients (and the revenue) or helping to orient a new therapist feels like a burden rather than a privilege. Even once the orientation process is underway, someone still has to fill in for the therapist who left, and you may find yourself begging staff members to pick up more hours or to cover more undesirable weekend and evening hours. Furthermore, your budget changes as you pay overtime for coverage on top of the salary of the new person being oriented, and you must absorb the hit to your revenue budget from not being able to bill for the therapy you don't have the staff to cover.

Staff in, staff out

As I was heading to work on the long commute one morning, all I could think about was how to find people to fill the three empty therapy slots for the skilled nursing facility located on our hospital campus. With one of my best therapists on the inpatient rehab unit leaving at the end of the month, and continual turnover problems in the outpatient therapy clinic, revenue was going to be down, physician complaints were going to go up, and the rest of the therapy staff was going to be physically and emotionally stretched.

I tried to concentrate on the drive, but my mind kept reverting back to the therapists I had lost in the past year. For each one, I kept asking myself, "What could I have done differently? Did they leave because of me, the organization, coworkers, or another reason? Would administration think I was the cause of therapists walking out the door?"

I know it was not a financial issue, as our salaries and benefits were very competitive. I dreaded the thought of the time I would have to spend going through advertising, applications, and interviews and all the stresses that go along with that process.

I promised myself that this time, things would be different; this time, I would not wait for people to tell me they wanted to leave. Instead, I would find a way to identify what I could do to keep them. For those who are still on staff with me, I would create a process I could use to work with them to ensure that they don't become a new statistic in the revolving door of therapy staff.

New therapy managers often have not been given the education, tools, and resources to manage recruitment and retention. Many organizations now realize the important role you play, not only in retention, but also in the likelihood that your staff members will recommend their place of employment to others. This book will provide you with resources and will guide you in using leadership skills to embrace the concept that you are the number one therapy recruiting officer for the organization.

Changing perceptions

The first step is to be realistic. You may need to change your attitudes and perceptions regarding keeping and recruiting talented staff. If any of the following thoughts are still in the back of your mind, make an attitude adjustment before you can hope to find success with your recruitment and retention strategies:

- "What more do they want from me? They're getting paid for what they do."

- "In my day, we were just grateful to get the job we wanted."

- "I'm getting really tired of 'making nice' just to keep people from leaving."

- "This new generation expects so much from us, but they are the first to say no to working a weekend or holiday shift."

These are the realities of rehab and therapy practice today. We are once again cycling through a therapy shortage, even if some areas of the country are experiencing more challenges than others. Our work force of baby boomers is getting older and retirement is very much on the horizon, and the new, young professionals are from a generation that has different values and expectations regarding their job. The role of the therapy manager has changed—you are more of a leader now than ever before.

Therapy managers play a key role

Realize the importance of your leadership role. You can find a way to ensure that the revolving door moves only when you want it to. You can embrace the research and evidence about work environments and how they directly affect the staff's perceptions. If money is the only thing people want, why do so many healthcare professionals, including therapists, report being dissatisfied with where they work, the resources available, and the managers to whom they report?

One of the most commonly uttered phrases in the healthcare tradition is "that's how we've always done it," but it is time to go ahead and break tradition. It is time to embrace new processes that will reap benefits not only for therapy staff, but also for patient care. You are taking a giant step forward as you embrace the contents of this book.

Chapter 2

Developing therapy managers and leaders

Administration can support and retain the therapy manager

Hospitals, nursing homes, clinics, and other healthcare organizations devote much time and effort to retention at the staff level, but they have forgotten the importance of retaining the middle manager. We have neglected to give adequate attention, nurturing, and support to the very people we hope will retain the therapists we recruit. An organization's recruitment and retention goals need to include the leaders who oversee the therapy staff.

Therapy managers' challenges

Administrators may view therapy managers as leaders who should not need hand-holding to want to stay in their jobs, but it is important for them to put themselves in the shoes of today's healthcare personnel, particularly therapy managers. In many facilities, managers face daily struggles to manage their workloads and support their limited staffs. We must make it a priority to support this vital group of employees and meet their professional and personal desires.

Promotion without training

Part of the challenge is that many therapy managers and leaders are selected for their positions based on their clinical skills, rather than on their leadership capabilities. We cannot expect people to stay and excel in positions for which they have no skills or training.

On the other end of the spectrum are those managers with appropriate leadership experience who accept positions. You are relieved to finally fill open positions, so you return to focus on your own job responsibilities. The new managers have the qualifications for the roles, have performed them well elsewhere, and will, you hope, ask for help or support if they need it. Such misperceptions can result in new managers who are unhappy because they sense a lack of administrative support. Imagine being a newly hired manager in a facility where you do not yet have a feel for the processes, the systems, or the team. Your new staff will test you to see how you measure up, the medical staff may not cooperate, and you'd like to fit in with your peer group, but no formal introductions were made through your administrative leader, so now you feel isolated and unprepared. Would you want to hang around through the 90-day probationary period?

Establish goals and expectations

Leadership development plays a vital role in the success and satisfaction of leaders, and it will directly affect the retention of all, not just the newly hired. Although retention efforts should focus on both new and seasoned managers, how you approach your retention efforts will, at times, be directed by a new manager's length of employment within the organization.

Tips for developing therapy leaders

The following tips should prove helpful for developing therapy leaders:

- Have senior administrators allot a specific time for retention efforts related to mid-level managers.

- Engage supervisors and managers in discussions to gain input on their individual requirements as they relate to professional development and personal needs.

- Identify the particular skills that supervisors and managers need to enhance their productivity and improve patient outcomes in their areas of responsibility. Provide the resources for them to attain these skills.

- Clarify and define success in their role from both your perspective and theirs. Reward this success on their performance evaluation.

- Schedule ongoing formal and informal communication opportunities between the new therapy manager and his or her direct supervisor.

Orienting the new manager

Regardless of where you are in a work relationship with the managers who report to you, there are important points to consider.

Sink or swim

Dave was hired two years ago as the therapy manager for a 35-bed inpatient rehabilitation facility in a large community medical center. He had four years of similar management experience at another inpatient rehab facility in a different state. Because of his previous experience, Dave was simply put through the hospital orientation program and then was off and running. As his administrator, you find yourself not only frustrated with complaints about him, but also disappointed in his inability to make things happen.

You schedule a meeting with Dave to share your concerns and to determine whether it is best for him to continue in this role. At the meeting, you discover not only that Dave is unhappy with his position, but also that he has put out feelers for openings at another facility across town. You ask him why he didn't come to you about this sooner and whether anything in particular is making him feel the need to leave.

Realize that both you and Dave perceive his role from two completely different perspectives. Without regular ongoing communication, both of you will continue to have misperceptions about what to expect.

Determine the accuracy of the job description

Is there a job description in writing that clarifies expectations? The job description may have been written several years ago and may not reflect the current issues that require the manager's oversight. Review the job description with the manager annually.

Identify management and leadership skills

Develop a process to identify a new manager's basic knowledge of management and leadership skills. Include terminology related to fiscal issues and formulas to calculate staffing and budget needs. This assessment will provide a work frame in which to develop goals and identify the manager's supportive and educational needs. (See Figure 2.1 for a sample assessment tool to measure new managers' knowledge/skills.)

Figure 2.1 | New-manager foundation knowledge/skills assessment

Please rate your level of comfort in independently performing the following functions/tasks:

1 = I have no experience with this

2 = I have a little experience, but I will need guidance

3 = I have some experience, but I will need a resource to go to the first few times

4 = I feel very comfortable with this, but I prefer that you check it the first time

5 = I can independently perform this

Please rate your level of comfort in independently performing the following functions/tasks:	
1 = I have no experience with this	1 2 3 4 5
2 = I have a little experience, but I will need guidance	1 2 3 4 5
3 = I have some experience, but I will need a resource to go to the first few times	1 2 3 4 5
4 = I feel very comfortable with this, but I prefer that you check it the first time	1 2 3 4 5
5 = I can independently perform this	1 2 3 4 5
1. Joint Commission/CARF/Medicare regulations	
Knowledge of those that apply to the clinical areas for which you are responsible	1 2 3 4 5
Ability to interpret standards	1 2 3 4 5
Knowledge of resources available to implement new standards	1 2 3 4 5
2. Quality assurance	
Ability to identify indicators for improvement processes	1 2 3 4 5
Ability to determine which processes require improvement	1 2 3 4 5
Knowledge of techniques to involve staff members in the improvement process	1 2 3 4 5
Knowledge of relating performance improvement to Joint Commission requirements	1 2 3 4 5
3. Fiscal responsibilities	
Productivity reporting and analysis	1 2 3 4 5
Understand budgeting terms and processes	1 2 3 4 5
Ability to relate month-to-date numbers to year-to-date figures	1 2 3 4 5
4. Technology skills	
Ability to use facility custom software and Microsoft programs	1 2 3 4 5
Working knowledge of electronic medical records and scheduling	1 2 3 4 5
Knowledge of Internet resources	1 2 3 4 5
5. Human resources	
Feel comfortable managing conflict on the unit	1 2 3 4 5
Understand facility and regulatory rules regarding termination and hiring	1 2 3 4 5
Ability to interview effectively	1 2 3 4 5
Knowledge of recruiting resources	1 2 3 4 5

Establish goals

Set goals to help managers see their accomplishments and allow you to feel their progress as leaders. This will also allow them to feel they are accomplishing something. (See Figure 2.2 for suggested goals.)

Figure 2.2 | Goals worksheet

Goals for new manager: Greg. Review progress with Greg at meeting on _____ (insert date).

1. Learn productivity system and be able to adjust budget and scheduling month ending _____ _____ (insert date).
2. Meet with CFO/financial officer to review revenue and expense budget process for the rehab department.
3. Meet with medical director of the rehab unit to initiate collaborative efforts regarding patient outcomes.
4. Draft outline of 12–24-month staff recruiting plan.

Rationale: Creating goals for all managers helps them to stay focused and to feel that they are accomplishing things that matter.

Provide support from peers

Assign all new managers a mentor from their peer group. Does the new manager have a hotline or other resource that he or she can access and with which the manager can leave a message if he or she needs resources or advice on an employee issue? The last thing you want is managers spending time trying to resolve something on which another manager can immediately direct them.

The following scenarios would be well served by such a resource:

- "I can't get Information Systems to print me my monthly budget report—they keep telling me that managers don't get a copy."

- "I need to refer an employee to the employee assistance program, and I can't get the counselor to return my phone calls."

- "To whom can I refer a rehab tech employee who is interested in going to PTA school and is looking for some scholarship resources?"

Equip them with tools

Provide them with the tools and resources they need to be successful in their roles. Provide a resource/reference library with books that enhance leadership and management skills.

Offer support and perspective

Schedule one-on-one meetings regularly. Make sure you have reviewed the reasons for which previous managers have left, even if you disagreed with their perceptions of the situation. They may offer valuable insight into how you can support the new manager.

Providing support, guidance, and direction

When you explore retention issues for staff members at this level of responsibility, the administrative team must make time to ask the manager some key questions. This simple action sends a message that the manager's input is important and that his or her role is valued by the overall organization. Have them ask the following questions:

- What is the one thing this organization provides you that has the greatest impact on maintaining your employment here?

- When you talk with others about how satisfied you are with your job, what are the things we do that give you that feeling of satisfaction?

- What do you think are some of the reasons other managers have left?

- If you had the power to add one benefit, process, or system related to your position, what would it be?

We generally consider leadership development to be simply providing education, resources, and tools for the manager, but it also includes picking up clues about whether managers are so overwhelmed that they cannot function in their roles. For retention efforts to be successful there has to be a place for helping managers who feel they are in over their head. Be alert to some of the warning signs that a manager needs to be thrown a life preserver.

Don't assume that things will be better next week. Make the effort now to confront your concerns and get help and support for the manager. You may do so through your employee assistance program, some time off, or a combination of administrative support and setting new, more realistic expectations. Warning signs of stress may include:

- Appearing unhappy or tired, losing or gaining weight, and being unable to focus or take direction

- Being constantly unable to meet deadlines

- Frequently canceling meetings set up with one's own manager

- Exhibiting negative nonverbal behavior

- Staff members going to other managers or the administrative team with concerns

Professional development: Ensuring a return on your investment

Some of the efforts that organizations make to retain or recruit a rehab supervisor or manager are unsuccessful. To better understand why, review typical scenarios that reflect some of the challenges and obstacles getting in the way of your efforts.

High hopes vs. everyday realities

You invested registration fees, airline and hotel costs, and paid time away for Monica, your new rehab manager, to attend a national meeting for rehab administrators. She returned enthusiastic, rejuvenated, and full of ideas and new networking resources. Her outlook quickly changed, how- ever, when reality set in—she returned to find her desk buried under piles of mail and stacks of green-bar computer printouts, her inbox full of requests from staff members, and her e-mail and voice mail at maximum capacity.

Case study

Such situations suck the enthusiasm out of a midlevel manager. You should take this opportunity to help develop Monica's organizational skills prior to her attending the meeting. Share some helpful tips that you use daily to manage paper flow, phone calls, and other office tasks when you are away so that the conference remains a boon instead of becoming another headache.

For example, you can hold a quick, informal meeting in which you help Monica discuss her expectations of her workload upon her return and prepare ways to manage it. Offer ways for her to remotely pick up e-mail and phone calls at the end of each conference day. Also suggest that Monica:

- Delegate a senior therapy staff member who will follow up on priority concerns she identifies from e-mail and phone calls

- Work with another manager from her peer group so that each can cover for the other when away for periods of time

- Post her schedule for the staff prior to her departure

- Schedule a catch-up half-day or day when she returns to work in order to prioritize her next steps

The knowledge and new ideas that Monica obtained at a conference will be valuable to other managers in the rehab area, so have her share her experiences at a managers' meeting. Schedule a specific date for this presentation, and if the conference sells audiotapes, have Monica bring the one that reflects what she feels was the most pertinent information of the conference. Using such a medium encourages other managers to participate in ongoing professional development. Another benefit of sending Monica to the conference is that doing so sends her a message that her role is important—that the organization is willing to invest in her ongoing education and professional development.

Mentor the manager

Another way to support managers is to assign them a mentor. Typically, the mentor should come from within the manager's peer group and can be effective and supportive if administration considers the following:

- Mentor selection should not be based on tenure with the organization; rather, it should be based on skills, character, and support for the mission.

- Administrators should work with mentors to develop a written assessment tool to identify baseline knowledge of both newly hired and established managers.

- Administrators should never assume that all is going well with the mentor simply because they have not heard otherwise. Body language reveals things that managers may be uncomfortable discussing proactively, so meet with them regularly, in person, to hear their perception of how things are going.

Look below the surface

Is there a problem? Are things going well? On the surface, it appears so. But if you don't ask, you will never know. It's worth being cautious about how new managers are doing, as they may not want to share with you what is really happening.

Ineffective mentor

Juanita, PT, has been a rehab and therapy manager at the facility for more than 15 years. She is well liked by her staff, the medical staff respects her, and administration can always count on her for help with last-minute issues.

She has been assigned as a mentor to Hank, OT, who was hired as a rehab manager four months ago for a sister hospital. After seeing them work together and collaborate at meetings, you walk away feeling good about the match. You meet with Hank monthly to discuss issues related to his department, and it appears that he is easily becoming a part of the organization.

He also has shared with you that his family is well settled into the community and that his wife is working locally.

Case study

For example, if you provide Hank with an evaluation tool that he can use to review his mentor, he may not want to reflect any negative comments on a peer, especially in writing. Therefore, to find out how he is really doing, schedule a meeting in which the two of you can openly discuss the realities of his new position.

Juanita may be doing a fine job of offering support to Hank and teaching him, for example, how to prepare and analyze productivity reports and other such tasks. However, because she has held the position for so long and because this facility is the only place where she has been a manager, she has always done things a certain way, and it is a challenge for her to be aware of options.

These facts mean that when Hank wants to discuss new protocols, standards, or approaches to staff issues, he gets a common response from Juanita: "That is not how we do things around here." There may also be some subtle differences because Juanita is a PT and Hank is an OT, even though they both have the position of rehab manager.

Mentoring is not a one-way learning process—Juanita could learn something from Hank as well. Consider using some of the prompters on the manager follow-up sheet (see Figure 2.3) to help you get to the pertinent information when you have this discussion with a new manager.

Successful leadership development requires continual effort

Leadership development is not a one-stop process. For it to be successful, it must be ongoing, and there must be commitment to it from the top. Your commitment becomes evident through your actions, not through what you may say you will do. Therefore, have a process to ensure that you follow through on requests, issues, and other staff concerns. Doing so is vital to the perceptions of managers who feel that their employer cares about them and cares about what they need.

Figure 2.3 | Manager follow-up prompters

The following questions can be used for new and seasoned rehab management staff:

- Now that you have been here for a few months, do you feel that having _____ as a mentor has been helpful?

- Because we each have our own personal style of managing, do you feel you can be yourself freely at this point? What have you implemented/done in your area(s) that you realize other managers here are not doing?

- What has surprised you the most about this organization?

- What skills can we help you to learn by providing the resources for you to obtain them?

- Because I work with so many different managers, it is a challenge at times to know specifically what each of you needs from me regarding time and other support. What can I do or provide for you to help you in your job?

- Can you think of something we have expected of you as part of your job that was an unrealistic expectation?

Improving interview skills

Although selecting new staff members to add to the team is one of the most important roles that rehab supervisors and managers play in relation to recruitment and retention, their interview skills typically are not addressed. New managers often are assumed to have such skills when they do not. Therefore, an important part of developing new rehab managers is to help them acquire the skills to choose appropriate staff members.

For example, although rehab managers are under intense pressure to fill vacant positions, we need to move away from hiring people just because their licenses are clean and they can start right away. The pressure to fill slots can never be an excuse to hire just any person who appears qualified. Support managers in making decisions that benefit the entire facility when they choose not to hire particular individuals—the long-term effects on morale and patient safety are not worth the trial-and-error option of hiring individuals who are not right for the job or the situation.

Practical tips to improve hiring skills

Use leadership development to improve the interview and hiring process by educating managers and providing them with resources and tools to guide them through the interview. Do the following:

- Incorporate interview scenarios in your monthly management meetings

- Ask each supervisor and manager to bring to the meeting what he or she feels is the most effective question he or she can ask at an interview

- Provide reference materials that can help the new manager improve interview techniques and approaches

- Demonstrate the importance of hiring for character versus hiring for skill through your own interview techniques

- Work with all your managers to address interview options that involve the staff

- Provide the staff with sample questions that prompt prospective hires to verbalize their skills, rather than having them show a certification card

- Use representatives from the human resources department to educate new managers on liability concerns during the interview process, such as those related to equal employment opportunity laws

It is important to help the new therapy manager understand that decisions to hire or not to hire will directly affect retention of the staff members who are already on the team. Teaching and guiding them through a process to develop these skills will reveal to them that anyone can look good on paper, but being able to function within the team will be revealed only through skilled interviewing.

Strategies to make time for the staff

Almost all managers want to spend more time with their staff, but they have so many responsibilities that they may have trouble finding the time. This situation leaves the therapists in the clinic, or on the floor, with the perception that managers are too busy pushing papers in their offices to spend time with them and that they do not see what they have to deal with. Time management is always a popular topic at meetings for managers, and although therapists often get some training in this area, many people tend to go back to habits they are comfortable with. Unfortunately, these old habits are usually the obstacles that prevent managers from using their time effectively.

Manager's support vital to morale

When you talk with staff members about what makes them stay at their job, a common response is "my manager." Staff members are happy when they feel that their manager respects their contributions and makes time for them. Managers receive satisfaction when they know they are directly responsible for some of the successes in their areas.

All new rehab supervisors and managers must develop an understanding of staff perceptions and how staff members relate their importance in the overall picture to how much time their manager spends with them. Develop managers to understand this concept and then to ask themselves how they can change this perception. Many opportunities present themselves at your regular manager meetings, so consider this topic for discussion among the therapy manager peer group.

Now is also a good time to look at what you discuss at these meetings. Save the memo reading for another time, and focus on leadership development topics. Start the discussion with suggestions for the therapy manager to consider, such as the following

- Availability at different therapy locations (floors/buildings/units/clinics, etc.) and different times several times per week. This doesn't have to be a formal arrangement; just be available.

- Schedule to meet with a different staff person one day a week for coffee or sit with him or her at lunchtime. Preschedule and post this information so that the staff can look forward to it.

- Keep each staff person's particulars related to his or her personal life in your contact management system. When you make time to take someone aside and ask how his or her ill family member is doing, you show that you actually care.

- Set up a calendar that lists each staff member's birthday. At the beginning of the month, celebrate the staff members who have birthdays that month.

- Post dates and times when you will have an "open door" for anyone who needs to talk. Be sure to stagger the times so that all can benefit.

When considering ways to help managers and leaders with their staff's development, ask yourself how you may be affecting retention:

- Have you developed your own goals for each supervisor and manager that reports to you?

- How can you personally affect retention of supervisors and managers?

- Are you willing to change some of your unrealistic expectations of the supervisors and managers?

- Can you commit, every day, to demonstrating the very behavior, professionalism, and support of the mission that you expect to see from your leadership team of supervisors and managers?

- Are you willing to invest time and resources into creating effective processes that enhance the retention of the nurse managers?

You are in a pivotal position not only to develop the managers and the roles they play, but also to create processes that retain managers effectively. Those you successfully develop and retain are our administrative healthcare leaders of the future. Feel good about who is going to be leading the way tomorrow by developing the rehab leaders of today.

Chapter 3

Employee and family policies and programs

Create an environment of care, concern, and respect

A vital part of recruitment and retention is to create a work environment that is employee- and family-friendly. Before you can begin to develop these policies and programs, make sure you are working in a culture that acknowledges and demonstrates care and concern for collegial interests and welfare. Lead through example by interacting with each of your colleagues and peers in a respectful and positive manner at all times.

Encourage positive relationships by taking the time to listen to and learn about the people with whom you work. Know their life priorities and motivators. Learn their children's names and where they're going to school. Ask about their pets. Develop a "significant other" bulletin board, and allow staff members to bring photos for display. Include a key at the bottom, identifying the staff member and whether the photo is of a child, parent, partner, pet, or friend.

Treat each person as an individual

Be open-minded and don't make assumptions. When a colleague asks for a special scheduling need, don't respond with "we can't do that here." Discuss the positives and negatives, and if there are concerns, ask the person making the request to do some research. Be willing to explore new options.

Enliven people's days by posting motivational or inspirational quotes. Clip cartoons and humorous stories that you know relate to a colleague's interests. Begin or end staff meetings by asking everyone to share something positive they experienced in the past week.

Look for positive behaviors in your colleagues and tell them as soon as you can what you saw and how impressed you were with them. In addition, although it may be a more difficult task, talk with colleagues about behaviors you observe that need to be corrected. When a group is asked, "How many of you would inform a colleague that he or she has bad breath?" only a few will raise their hands. But when asked whether they would want a colleague to tell them if they had bad breath, almost everyone in the room raises his or her hand. This illustrates that almost all of us are approachable and willing to hear how we can improve, if that approach is done in a thoughtful, encouraging manner. The first step to improving coworker behavior can be daunting, but it is important to take it anyway.

Evaluate employee needs before creating policies

Although vacation, annual leave, health and dental insurance, and retirement planning have become standard benefits for most healthcare organizations, those seeking to meet the evolving needs of their employees and families should consider several additional benefits and programs.

How to judge employee needs

One of the key elements to success with any employee- or family-oriented program is to know the needs of staff members and their families. You can gather this data with a survey and simply hope that you get responses from the majority of people who have the greatest need, or you can use your best resource—the staff members who work with you. Form a committee made up of people who know the details and needs of staff members and their families.

Ensure diverse representation on the committee

The members of the committee or task force should include:

- Staff-level employees from various types of positions

- Employees from diverse age groups

- A balance of male and female employees

- The cultural diversity present in your staff

- Staff members who do and do not have a need for such programs

- Representatives from the midlevel management and top management groups

- Representatives from personnel or human resources

For workplace enhancement programs to be successful, they must have direct commitment and support from the organization. Both can be accomplished with a clear written statement from senior management that sends a message to all employees that the organization believes in the program and encourages staff members and their families to take advantage of what will be offered. Employees must believe the statement is sincere and not feel that they are just being pacified because staff members at the hospital down the road got a pay raise and they didn't.

Some tips to consider in helping the committee plan and develop programs include the following:

- Rotate members of the committee on an annual basis

- Have clear written objectives and a timeline for what you want them to accomplish

- Give them the resources they need to meet their goals

- Make sure that members of top management are available to sit in on meetings occasionally

- Require written policies that explain the qualifications for these programs

- Develop a process to evaluate the effectiveness of each program

- Collect data on how frequently each program is used

- Charge committee members with educating all of the managers about the programs, rules, policies, and so on before you enact any program

Promote the programs

The best employee- and family-friendly programs cannot help if no one accesses them. Therefore, start a marketing campaign for what you will be offering. Get the word out through word of mouth, e-mail notifications, newsletters, posters, brochures, mailings to employees' homes, and promotional activities at annual employee functions.

Employee assistance programs

Many organizations offer employee assistance programs, which may be as basic as offering a toll-free hotline for crisis issues or as extensive as counseling for parents and their teenage children.

Private companies offer these services to organizations that do not want to be involved in hiring and overseeing the staff that runs these programs. Some healthcare organizations want a more "hands-on" approach, so they hire staff and are involved with the specifics of the day-to-day operations. Note that the program's success will relate directly to how sure staff members are that the information is kept confidential.

You may want to consider options that include allowing employees to seek appointments on their own for referrals to private counselors. The program could offer monthly training on relationships, addictions, and other problem issues, and it even could help employees who are in financial turmoil and need temporary assistance. In addition, managers should be able to refer a staff member to receive counseling from the program's personnel, should he or she continue to display unacceptable behaviors.

The manager's role in promoting the employee assistance program

Employees in need of help or in a crisis within their family structure often forget that this service is available to them. Once they finish their orientation process, they tend not to hang on to handbooks and other brochures that explain benefits and free services. Therefore, management should step in to remind staff members of these types of services and consider offering them to employees as an option when behavior issues arise. Managers also must trust that the program is strictly confidential; otherwise, they will be unable to reassure the staff that it is.

Employee assistance programs may offer numerous benefits

With an active, reputable employee assistance program, your organization not only helps to retain valuable staff members, but also has a wonderful recruiting tool. With so many family challenges in today's world, there is nothing wrong with asking for professional help to get the family unit back on target.

Design your employee assistance brochures with targeted services that people feel comfortable talking about, instead of simply highlighting services for domestic violence victims and addictions. Although your employees need to know you offer all these services, the enticement for the program lies in services such as:

- Financial counseling

- Counseling for children, especially teenagers

- Classes on negotiating with teens, coping with teens, addressing eating disorders, and so on

- Marriage retreats

- Referrals for employees interested in adopting children

- Classes on managing time within the family

- Classes for children of divorced parents

On-site health clinics and wellness centers

Another employee and family program that can be of great assistance and can be perceived as a wonderful benefit is a health clinic. Such clinics operate during specific hours and days of the week and are good resources for staff members or their immediate family members for minor healthcare needs. Clinics deter employees from using the emergency room as a resource.

Wellness centers offer prevention advice

Another option is to have a wellness center that focuses on primary prevention. More organizations are helping employees maintain physical and emotional wellness by providing an on-site or off-site fitness center, a fitness trainer, a nutritional counselor, and wellness incentives.

Additionally, invest in your employees' health by working toward a no-lift or minimal-lift work environment. Investment in lift-assistive devices to prevent back and joint injuries can be recouped through savings in worker compensation and absenteeism reduction.

Offer a wide variety of benefit options

As well as vacation, medical, and dental benefits, consider offering employees a pretax benefit plan, which can provide a variety of pretax benefits through an employer-managed plan that can be created under U.S. federal tax law. Certain medical, child care, and adult care expenditures can be paid with these pretax dollars. Normally, a pretax portion of each paycheck is paid into a reimbursement account, and as eligible expenses are paid, the employee is reimbursed for them.

Some federal employees are allowed seven days in addition to annual or sick leave to serve as bone marrow or organ donors. Other organizations offer leave-sharing programs, whereby fellow employees can donate accumulated leave time to a colleague who may have exhausted his or her own allotment.

Some organizations provide stipends to assist employee families who are going through the adoption process. The employees are also granted maternal and paternal leave to promote mother–child and father–child bonding.

Some organizations even allow employees to bring pets to the workplace. Although that my not be possible in direct care settings, some hospitals are negotiating pet health insurance purchase plans and rates for their staff.

Flexible work arrangements

Be open to flexible work arrangements that will meet the needs of both your employees and your organization. By keeping an open mind and exploring different options, you can improve staff satisfaction and retention.[1]

Temporary part time: Some staff members may choose to always work part time, but consider options that allow full-time staff members to temporarily work part time. This option should be mutually agreed upon by the employee and the therapy manager, but it may be helpful on a short-term basis in times of personal or family crises, or even upon returning from a break.

Job-sharing: Allowing and encouraging job-sharing, where appropriate, will give part-time flexibility to staff members who want it. Under such an arrangement, full-time job responsibilities, duties, hours, and pay can be divided among two or more employees.

Consider nontraditional options

A variety of nontraditional options may also be considered.

Flextime: Flextime is becoming increasingly popular in the corporate world, and some hospitals and rehab clinics are successfully adapting the concept. Some facilities allow therapists with small children to begin work later in the morning so that they can drop their children off at school. They work through the day, and in the afternoon, they pick the children up from school, spend quality time with them and their significant other over dinner, and then return to work for a few additional hours. With care, you can develop a flextime policy that allows employees within a team or on an individual basis to choose their own start and finish times.

Compressed work weeks: Although some studies question the safety of working 12-hour shifts, many healthcare employees enjoy the ability to compress their workweek into three or four 12-hour days per week. Likewise, straight weekend or weekend-option schedules are attractive to some healthcare professionals. Consider a variety of workday schedules, such as 8, 10, and 12 hours, but analyze safety and quality indicators closely so as not to sacrifice either in the name of employee friendliness.

Schedules that coincide with school terms: Another option for employees with school-age children may be to create a work schedule that coincides with your local school term. The term is usually 9½ months with summers off, but it may be throughout the year if your schools use year-round schedules.

Telecommuting and teleworking: Although therapy is a direct care service, consider tasks that can be completed via computer or telecommunication links to your organization. There may be positions in which all or some of the hours can be completed from home.

Part-time therapist, part-time compliance specialist

Marianne, PT, is an orthopedic therapist who works in the hospital system's spine rehab clinic. She has four children under the age of six, and is finding it difficult to maintain her traditional 8 a.m.–4:30 p.m. job as a staff therapist.

During her annual evaluation, she asked to work part time so that she could better handle her child care needs. Her rehab manager came up with a proposition that would allow Marianne to continue full time. Marianne would work three days a week in the clinic, and two days she would telework as a compliance specialist for rehab. Marianne's telejob allowed her remote access to rehab medical records and current documentation. Marianne was responsible for reviewing rehab medical records for the hospital's 13 therapy locations. This is a win-win situation: The hospital provided a unique solution that allowed an experienced therapist to maintain full-time status, and the therapist was able to complete her compliance activities on a 24/7 basis.

Carry over leave time: Provide flexibility in allowing staff members to carry annual leave into the next calendar year. It should be mutually agreed upon by the manager and employee, but such an arrangement may be helpful in certain situations such as travel abroad.

Employment breaks: Some employees may be interested in taking longer breaks. Consider developing a policy that allows those who have been with you for longer than 12 months to be able to request up to a one-year employment break. Paid employment with another employer would not be taken during this period, and you would assure the individual that, upon return, a job of equal status within your organization would be provided. Personal reasons that might warrant interest in this benefit include a prolonged illness in the family, care of a parent, charity work, or world travel.

Self-scheduling: This option allows certain staff members to schedule their time based on parameters negotiated by their manager. It promotes satisfaction and autonomy among employees.

Phased retirement: This option allows older employees to retire gradually by reducing full-time hours over a period of years. As demand for healthcare professionals increases, some states are enacting policies to remove retirement penalties and work limits to allow qualifying employees to receive full retirement benefits and continue to work full time.

Programs that save employees time

Many of these programs ask: What can you do to make life easier for the employee? Anytime you can answer this question with a program or service, you have created a recruitment and retention tool.

Everyone wants more time, so help your employees find time for activities they value. Providing the following types of services gives employees more time with their families when they are not at work:

- The third Wednesday of each month staff members can call the local grocery store and reserve a complete cooked dinner, for a special price. They pick it up that day between specified hours.

- The local dry cleaner has an area in the hospital where staff members can leave their clothes for dry cleaning and pick them up the next workday. Payment is prearranged through the employee's credit card, so the facility does not have to deal with financial transactions.

- Make arrangements with the local optical shop for all employees and their immediate family members to receive a discount on eye exams and frames or contact lenses.

- A local oil change company picks up employees' cars from the parking lot and returns them after an oil change. Payment can also be handled through the employee's credit card.

Other employee- and family-friendly programs

In addition to the programs mentioned, your organization can provide other employee- and family-friendly programs.

Child care: Some healthcare organizations provide on-site child care services, and others negotiate rates and openings with local child care agencies. Having child care options can benefit a large portion of your staff, and worker satisfaction increases when parents are happy with their child care arrangements.

Adult care: You may be surprised at the number of employees who are primary care providers for their parents or older relatives. These employees may be more interested in adult care services as a benefit.

Help with partner's employment search: Consider providing assistance with an employment search of a spouse or partner of a candidate or current employee with a partner opportunities program.

Seminars: Make an effort to meet other needs of your employees by providing "brown-bag" or evening seminars on a variety of family issues. Survey your staff to determine their interests and what they may find most helpful or interesting.

Showing employees that you value them

Make a commitment to demonstrate to employees that they are valued.

The power of everyday surprises

Regardless of age and occupation, many people love surprises. It is the element of the unexpected and the fact that someone took the time to think of it that make it special.

If you develop leadership skills in your managers by teaching this concept, you empower them with simple employee-friendly ideas. The size of the surprise does not necessarily relate to how happy it makes the person on the receiving end. Surprises do not have to be attached to rewards, although they can and should be when appropriate. Surprises are not simply about celebrating a birthday in the department.

Simple surprises

Consider how the following simple surprises can make employees feel valued:

- The manager takes the caseload of the therapist who has the longest tenure (or any other designation that you choose). After the manager reviews the caseload for the day, the therapist is given the day off with pay and a Starbucks card thanking him or her for his or her commitment to the patients and the organization.

- At the end of the day, top-level management are stationed outside with buckets of soap, sponges, and hoses to wash employees' cars before they go home.

- The CEO of the organization calls a rehab manager in the morning and invites him or her to lunch that day to brainstorm and share ideas about improving patient care.

What employees really want

In *Love 'Em or Lose 'Em: Getting Good People to Stay,* authors Beverly L. Kaye and Sharon Jordan-Evans surveyed 12,000 people, identifying 20 reasons why they remained at a company. Here is a list of the top eight answers:

1. Exciting work and challenges

2. Career growth, learning, and development

3. Working with great people

4. Fair pay

5. Supportive management/good boss

6. Being recognized, valued, and respected

7. Benefits

8. Meaningful work and making a difference

These results remind us that although employee- and family-friendly programs are important, they should not be developed to replace other vital qualities employees need from their employers, such as trust, ethics, training, and development.

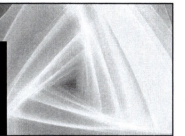

Developing professional models of care

Professional models of care promote retention

Professional models of patient care delivery are constantly changing and improving. Employees in any profession want to work in an organization that provides a great product or service, and therapists in healthcare settings are no different. They want to work in settings that provide great patient care.

Health consumers have high expectations for healthcare delivery systems, and it is only right that they should expect safe, quality, individualized care. To address patient expectations for quality care, healthcare systems must develop care delivery systems that encourage, support, and practice autonomy and decision-making for therapists.

Allow rehab therapists to practice to the best of their ability

Employers should construct and implement systems that allow therapists to practice within their full scope of practice. Practice policies and procedures should be based on discipline-specific practice standards and evidence-based outcomes. Employers must recognize, through support of clinical research and therapist-directed care improvements, that therapists contribute knowledge and expertise to quality patient care and patient outcomes.

Strong rehab leadership

Managers play an integral role in creating a culture of quality care and workplace improvement. Therefore, hire qualified, well-prepared therapy managers capable of fulfilling management functions and roles. Provide support and encouragement for managers through programs and policies. Develop a comprehensive list of manager competencies, including such basics as:

- Adherence to ethics and practice standards

- Effective communication and interpersonal skills

- Conflict resolution

- Decision-making

- Problem-solving

- Delegation

- Human resources management

- Financial and budget management—including regulatory compliance with CMS and state requirements

- Provision of staff evaluations and performance appraisals

- Internal and external marketing

Also inquire about their abilities to demonstrate broader manager competencies, such as:

- Caring for self, patients, and staff

- Implementing quality improvement processes

- Practicing negotiation and conflict resolution

- Promoting collaborative interdisciplinary relationships

- Ensuring patient safety

- Developing staff

- Devising systems and administrative theories

- Monitoring financial resources

- Monitoring human resources

- Being politically savvy

- Conducting research utilization and implementation

- Developing policies

- Conducting strategic planning

Help managers look critically at their skills and develop a program for self-improvement. You'll want to groom therapy staff members to help with operational functions whenever possible to allow managers to focus on these broader management and leadership skills.

In a culture constantly seeking improvements, managers do not only need to manage, they also need to lead. As a manager, you must manage resources and work with your staff to remove barriers to quality care, but as a leader, you must improve your self-knowledge regarding areas of strength and areas you can improve. Thus, becoming a leader involves developing strategic skills that help position your department for a successful future. It includes taking risks, incorporating creative ways of group problem-solving, and improving patient care. Leadership requires you to develop coaching, mentoring, and grooming skills. It includes shaping and sharing compelling messages that inspire and encourage staff members to provide organizational policy development, strategic planning, and operational decision-making in an effort to improve patient care. In a professional work environment, therapy managers and leaders make sure that rehabilitation is an integral part of any organizational committee that governs policy and operational decision-making.

Therapist-directed patient care

Establish departmental and organizational cultures that encourage and foster therapist-directed care. In professional practice models, therapists make autonomous decisions within their scopes of practice and control care-delivery standards in the practice environment. They establish practice standards, set patient care goals, make decisions concerning managing and monitoring patient care, and measure patient outcomes. Work with your staff and administration to develop and implement policies that mandate professional therapist authority to control the practice by developing therapy practice policies.

Review your organizational structure periodically with the staff, and discuss the impact of communication and decision-making at the point of care. Use staff meetings to share examples of decisions made by therapists in the rehab unit that directly influenced positive patient outcomes. You might even begin staff meetings by asking the staff to share how their decisions made a difference in patient care and improved satisfaction. You also can ask them to share a decision that made them feel uneasy or uncertain, and either confirm their actions or ask fellow staff members to discuss how they would have reacted to that type of situation. Reaffirm your commitment to decision-making at the point of care, and assess staff needs for continuing education programs that promote self-development in decision-making and leadership skills.

Having therapists participate in shared governance structures and councils encourages therapists to be autonomous and accountable decision-makers at the point of care. It also encourages them to practice fully within the scope of individual therapists' professional standards of practice.

Adequate and appropriate staffing

Adequate staffing is another component of professional care models. The adequacy of facility staffing, particularly in the form of therapist productivity ratios, has received much attention in recent years. The goal is to provide cost-effective, quality staff and staffing patterns. Ultimately, staffing decisions must be made by therapists and managers on a basis that accounts for revenue as well as expense.

Make sure you are using the right healthcare professional with the correct competencies for providing quality patient care. Plan your staffing patterns to maintain an adequate number of qualified therapists, therapy assistants, and rehab techs to meet the therapy requirements for the individual units and clinics that you are staffing.

Staffing options

Always adjust staffing patterns as patient demands change, and encourage employees to make suggestions concerning staffing options. Ask for their thoughts on times when they feel that they may be understaffed or overstaffed. If you are in a locale that is subject to part-time residents during certain times of the year, staffing may need to adjust to the flux of patient referrals during those times.

However you make your decisions, promote teamwork and consider strategies that extend the present work force, such as making support services and management therapy personnel available to help therapists meet evolving patient care demands. For example, if your staff feels that therapy services are understaffed due to multiple new patients and the need for screening evaluations, try assigning a therapist to work a schedule that focuses on new-patient screenings for potential program admission.

Develop a formal system of evaluation

Develop a formal system for evaluating the effects of staffing patterns. This is also requirement of The Joint Commission, and skill mix on patient outcomes. For example, develop a productivity tool that therapy supervisors use to rate the adequacy of staffing for each clinic and service area. However you measure it, make sure that staffing is consistently adequate to provide quality patient care.

Quality improvement processes

Professional work environments are committed to quality improvement, evidence-based practice, and quality patient care. Ensure that therapists are incorporated into organizational quality improvement committees, and provide them with continuing education, coaching, and role-modeling in research and evidence-based practice. Identify expected outcomes with benchmarks for acceptable quality service, and conduct quality outcome measurements to determine your progress. Traditionally, quality improvement processes have been applied almost exclusively to improving patient care, but be sure to apply the same processes to improving your workplace culture and environment.

Report your results

Provide quality care outcomes or indicators to your quality management and quality improvement committees to recommend practice improvements and address concerns. Establish a utilization review system to conduct analysis and correction of patient care and safety concerns and issues.

Providing interdisciplinary forums will encourage discussion of collaborative strategies for improving patient care and eliminating duplication of services among disciplines. Develop processes for immediate reporting of unsafe or inadequate care, and implement a system by which employees can recognize and reward colleagues who deliver quality patient care.

Building competent teams

Helping your staff with self-improvement can be as simple as asking one of your experienced staff members to initiate and lead a journal club. The leader of the club selects an article, makes copies for distribution, and has members of the club meet for 15–30 minutes to discuss the findings that apply to your work area. Such a club is a great strategy for applying the latest research findings to the practice setting, and it helps your staff to keep up with the latest skills and competencies. This can also be done as a "lunch and learn," and pizza or submarine sandwiches can be ordered in.

Valuing colleagues

Help employees understand the value of individual contributions to quality patient care. Discuss the team effort required and establish a culture of mutual valuing and respect. Help your staff members understand that each individual contributes specific skills and competencies and that each is important.

Develop a "We Care" rather than a "Me Care" patient safety and quality care culture. Help the staff understand that the delivery of quality care requires more than just holding oneself accountable for doing the right things. It also requires healthcare professionals to make sure our healthcare systems help all personnel to do the right things, leaving little or no room for error. Help staff members to develop policies and systems that encourage them to deliver safe, quality, ethical, and error-free care.

With the stress of a healthcare work environment and the diverse personalities, opinions, and competencies among personnel, conflict is inevitable. Therefore, develop formal processes for dealing with it. Establish behavior standards or a professional conduct code that includes zero tolerance for rude or demeaning behavior, and make sure the staff is aware of the policies. These policies should require immediate counseling by managers or supervisors for internal personnel and by the administrator or CEO for external personnel (e.g., physicians, paramedics, or visitors). A professional code of conduct should be held to all employees, medical staff, volunteer staff, and vendors.

Measuring benefits of professional models of care

Using components and principles of professional models of care can improve staff retention and quality patient care. Doing so makes healthcare safer, as demonstrated by lower error rates, and improves quality of care delivery, as evidenced by higher patient satisfaction scores. Another benefit of incorporating professional models of care is that the retention of healthcare personnel improves through lower turnover rates, lower vacancy rates, and higher retention rates. In addition, staff morale is improved and demonstrated by higher employee satisfaction scores.

Implementing quality improvement systems

The need for quality improvement systems

Quality improvement processes and systems dramatically improve patient care outcomes. It is in the best interest of every hospital and healthcare delivery system to develop patient care standards and systems that consistently improve patient safety and care. It is also in the best interest of healthcare employers to implement quality workplace improvement processes and systems to create a workplace culture and environment that attracts and retains excellent healthcare professionals.

In such a quality workplace, therapy managers, administration, and staff members support a quality work environment. They develop standards and systems for sustaining a quality work-place. Therapy leaders receive essential data and information, have authority and account-ability, and are integrally involved in decisions that affect the workplace environment.

First steps in developing quality improvement systems

When beginning a program, first ensure that administrator, manager, and staff performance evaluations include the criteria for creating a quality workplace. Also incorporate workplace improvement criteria into employee performance appraisals.

Establish clear goals for workplace excellence. Develop systems that not only meet Occupational Safety and Health Administration standards, but also exceed regulatory workplace safety standards. In a service-delivery profession, your employees are among your most valuable assets.

Create a workplace environment committee

Include all staff members from representative departments on committees responsible for ensuring worker safety and illness prevention. For example, form a committee to identify and make recommendations concerning workplace improvements or establish a workplace environment council. One of the group's responsibilities might be to evaluate the purchase of products or systems that promote employee safety.

Although ensuring patient and employee safety may be a basic goal of these committees, a loftier goal would be to create a workplace environment that fosters employee wellness, engagement, and commitment. Therefore, ask the committee to develop strategies that promote the physical, emotional, spiritual, professional, and social wellness of your staff. It could make recommendations concerning meaningful work and develop policies and programs that promote employee engagement and commitment—and an engaged and committed employee is a loyal employee.

A workplace environment committee will focus on prevention strategies to decrease illness, injury, stress, and accidents among employees. Consider placing at least one member on the human resources committee that reviews compensation and benefits.

Committees also can collect data on employee satisfaction and make evidence-based recommendations based upon employees' needs and interests. The committee might recommend a no-lift or minimal-lift policy; rehab staff can be integral in providing information leading to the support for this decision, as well as how to best implement it. They also might develop an initiative to prevent workplace violence and provide support for employees who experience violence. This committee could set safety and security quality improvement goals and conduct root cause analyses on incidents involving employees.

Quality workplace improvement principles

Several principles are helpful when considering quality workplace improvements.

Focus on the employee

The ultimate customers of any healthcare delivery organization are the patients, but the most important internal customers are your employees. If you care for your employees, they will care for your patients. You cannot deliver patient care without healthcare professionals, and each has unique needs, wants, and motivators. Thus, just as hospitals and healthcare systems have established systems and processes to deliver individualized, customized patient care, they must develop systems and processes to provide individualized, customized employee care.

Understand the work culture as systems and processes

When you look at the complete picture of a workplace culture and environment, it can seem incomprehensible and overwhelming. Therefore, take one thing at a time, and analyze specific systems and processes. For example, identify communication processes that occur among the staff, such as therapist to therapist or therapist to rehab tech. Talk with your staff to ascertain what needs to be improved first.

Also, seek to improve collaboration among and between staff members, on different work schedules, units and clinics, and so on. Focus your efforts to improve one system or process at a time, and begin with the areas that are causing the most dissatisfaction among your staff. This will help you develop a work force code of professional conduct.

Practice teamwork

Include as many of your staff members in the improvement discussions as you can. Ask for their thoughts, ideas, and assistance in putting improvements in place. Each has a vested interest in improving the workplace, and because each is a frontline employee, each can contribute significant insight and expertise. As a manager, define parameters or limits for workplace improvement discussions, but make sure that you use their helpful recommendations and suggestions. Remind your staff that workplace improvements should benefit the entire healthcare team. Expect to allow "nonproductive" time for staff participation.

Focus on the use of data

Help the staff to understand the power of data. When a particular issue is raised, ask the staff to document it for a week or so to determine how often the type of incident actually occurs. For example, if linens are late arriving to the outpatient clinic, have the therapy supervisors document how often this occurs before you decide whether to take corrective action. If the therapy staff reports an increase in belligerent visitors, ask them to document the time of day or the circumstances under which this occurs. Upon analysis, you might find that the incidents are occurring during a certain patient's clinic time, so you can look at strategies to decrease some of the chaos that occurs at that time. You'll want your workplace improvements to be evidence-based, and data provides that evidence.

Key steps to improvement

Establishing where to begin your quality workplace improvement is the first challenge.

Begin with what's causing the most pain

Identify what's causing your staff the most concern or pain. Ask staff members to develop a list of workplace issues they would like to see improved, and help them to prioritize and select issues to be addressed. Be aware that if your staff has not participated in this type of process, you may want to begin with a few issues in which you can demonstrate quick successes. For example, instead of beginning by trying to improve employee parking, begin by contracting with a local dry cleaner to provide pick-up and delivery service. Once they have a few successes under their belt, you can help them tackle more challenging workplace issues, such as improving therapy–nursing relations or collaboration with other units. Use data from your employee satisfaction survey, exit interviews, or staff discussions to identify workplace improvement issues.

Develop a workplace improvement committee

Although retention is everyone's responsibility, you'll need to establish a committee or council to focus on workplace improvements. Some organizations use a recruitment and retention committee, which usually focuses on recruitment and retention strategies, but the workplace committee discussed earlier is often a better option because its goal is to provide a quality workplace, which would enhance both recruitment and retention.

Collect and analyze workplace data and information

It is imperative that you collect a variety of workplace data, and at times you'll want to implement research and outcomes studies. Establish systems that provide constant feedback from your employees. Don't collect data for the sake of collecting data. Collect only what you need, but give thoughtful consideration to data sources that will help you identify workplace improvement trends and issues. Use evidence-based decision-making to identify areas for change and improvement, and allow enough to analyze the data and information.

Exit interviews

When employees leave your organization, collect exit interview data in a consistent, anonymous manner so that they can tell you the real reasons they're leaving. Most employees do not want to decrease their chances of being rehired if needed, so make sure they feel that they can be truthful in their responses. Managers should not administer the exit interview, but instead should have it administered by computer, conducted in the human resources office, or outsourced to a third party.

Performance appraisals

Annual performance appraisals are an ideal time to collect employee ideas on workplace improvements. You're probably already using performance appraisals to determine competency training needed for your unit. Consider including competencies that relate to interpersonal communication and interdisciplinary collaboration. You also might ask each employee to share the top three things he or she likes most about working on your unit and the top three things he or she likes least about working there. If you tally your responses, you'll get an idea of what features are valued by your staff and are working, and you'll make sure the needs of your staff continue to be met. An analysis of the items they like least will help you focus on areas for workplace improvements.

Incremental interviews

Incremental interviews are used when you learn that an employee is considering leaving your unit and you'd like to retain him or her. This interview can provide helpful information for workplace improvements, but its main focus is to prevent a quality staff member from leaving. You certainly can ask what the employee likes or does not like about working there, but the main question you'll ask is "What can we do to keep you here?" You'll also want to spend time identifying the employee's career goals and discussing options you can provide on your unit to help him or her achieve those goals.

Individualized measurements

Sometimes you may want to conduct individualized measurements of specific workplace issues. For example, you may wish to evaluate employee levels of stress. Particularly when the patient census is high, measure levels of employee stress and identify stressors in the work environment. You also might determine the types of strategies that help relieve stress for your staff.

Appreciative inquiry

Collect data through appreciative inquiry by asking your staff to identify what your organization is doing right, rather than what it is doing wrong. Although it can be helpful to make improvements in an organization, appreciative inquiry helps to identify what's working well. Rather than focusing on what is wrong with a system, this theory advises organizations to focus on strengths and capabilities to achieve improvement goals. Ask your staff to share workplace improvement success stories. If you're focusing on improving interpersonal communication, have staff members share communication behaviors they observed during the workday that promoted positive outcomes. The goal is to verbalize positive behaviors that you would like other staff members to replicate. Appreciative inquiry has helped several healthcare systems improve patient satisfaction, and it holds great promise to do the same for employee satisfaction.

Focus groups

Bring together groups comprising 8–10 staff members to focus on specific issues. If you're attempting to develop strategies to retain mature, experienced therapists, invite a group of "baby-boomer" therapists who are 50 and older from different areas to identify incentives, benefits, and work improvements that would encourage them to work longer. Be willing to provide flextime for your 50+ staff. They might also provide insight into the types of work incentives that can attract older therapists who are willing to work part time, or take a position on a temporary basis. You might decide to hold a focus group for several different therapy service areas if you are in a large healthcare system.

To get consistent group responses, develop a script with questions to use with each group. Response data and information from the groups can be documented, tallied, and analyzed to identify priority issues and strategies. If you have a work force management and development department use those staff members to conduct the focus groups rather than the therapy director.

Employee satisfaction monitoring

More and more employers understand the need to monitor employee satisfaction. Healthcare delivery is an employee-intensive service, so it is especially vital for employers to retain staff. Some healthcare organizations are outsourcing employee satisfaction surveys and data analysis. Others have developed an in-house employee satisfaction survey tool. Either is fine, as long as it provides unbiased trends and findings pertaining to employee satisfaction. Use employee satisfaction findings to help identify areas and issues for workplace improvement.

Considering change and improvement

Upon reviewing findings and trends from multiple sources of workplace data, or after hearing a workplace issue verbalized by numerous staff members, you will begin to think, "Maybe we should do something about this." It's at that moment that you must consider whether it is worth the effort to make the change or improvement, or whether it is better to maintain the status quo. Here's a process that will help you make that decision.

Step 1: Identify what must improve

This step may sound redundant, but you must determine what needs to improve. For example, let's say that your employee satisfaction survey identifies that staff members feel therapy–nurse interactions need major improvement. As a rehab manager, you may already hold insight into the particulars of the issue, and the employee satisfaction findings only validate your earlier suspicions. But let's say you had no idea that therapy–nurse interactions needed improvement. To determine what actually needs to improve, you might talk with some of your therapists or the nurses to gather more in-depth information. You might even hold one focus group with therapists and one with nurses in order to gather input. Are the negative interactions coming from one-on-one discussions? Does it relate to calling nurses every morning to remind them that patients must be in therapy on time? Or is it a professional trust issue? (Can we really trust the nursing staff to conduct passive range of motion?) Your goal is to determine what must improve.

Step 2: Analyze and understand the problem

Help your workplace improvement group to analyze and understand the problem. Make sure they have all available data and information, and allow time to discuss, dissect, and process problem scenarios. Ask them to identify specific systems and processes that require improvement, and require them to recommend desired outcomes.

Step 3: Consider and develop

Consider what changes will improve the problem, and develop strategies that accomplish your desired outcomes. Brainstorming can be a useful technique for developing strategies. Ask your employees to blurt out any ideas, no matter how wacky or far out, in a 10-minute period. Ask one staff member to write the ideas on a flip chart as they are suggested. The only rule is that no one is allowed to judge another staff member's idea. After the ideas are documented, encourage the group to select the top three strategies for further discussion and consideration.

Step 4: Test and implement

Consider testing your thoughts and recommendations to see whether they yield improvements. Once your staff has determined a best option, develop plans to test the strategy to see whether it provides desired outcomes. Then you and your staff can decide whether to abandon, modify, or permanently implement the solution.

A model for testing change in the workplace

Plan

Develop a plan for the change. Consider the impact of the change on patient care, workplace, and employee outcomes. Identify methods for measuring your desired outcomes. Make sure that you and your staff communicate the pilot test for change to all employees affected by the change.

Pilot-test

Establish start and completion dates, and test the change. Collect data and document the results of the change. Continue to monitor the outcomes.

Analyze results

Review data, and realistically evaluate positive or negative effects of the change. Verify your methods and results to make sure they are accurate.

Implement change

Modify, abandon, or implement the change. Develop a process to monitor outcomes consistently and consider implementing the improvement in your workplace.

Identify a successful workplace quality improvement initiative

Peer resources are invaluable in sparking ideas and offering insight in systems that work well. A suggested activity is to identify several programs that you and your staff perceive to be excellent. Contact your peer at those programs and open a discussion regarding workplace improvements in rehab. From your discussions, identify the rehab facility that has implemented a successful work-place improvement that you would most like more information about. Your goal is to further study the workplace improvement program that you have identified. This can include a "field trip" to the facility, phone interviews with key staff members involved in the process, a review of program reports, and so on.

To allow for successful, long-term change you should seek approval from administration. This is especially true in a productivity-driven rehabilitation department. It's best to set hours aside for the improvement team to participate on the committee and gauge employee satisfaction.

Ensuring interdisciplinary collaboration

Case study

Lack of collaboration breeds discontent

The therapists in the nursing home's skilled rehab unit have worked together for several years. They feel a strong presence of team support among their peers and are encouraged by a rehab manager who uses effective strategies to enhance their work environment. So, why are they unhappy? The nursing home system has negotiated a new contract for rehab administrative services with a larger group from the medical center about an hour away, and new people have entered the environment. What was a peaceful workplace has become a battlefield.

The preceding situation is a classic example of a noncollaborative environment. The new rehab administrative group showed up at the nursing home with unrealistic expectations of the existing staff, and the existing rehab therapy staff was not involved in the process of changing to a new administrative team. The facility took no steps to get the new relationship off to a good start, and the result was an environment filled with difficult scenarios.

First, the new administrative group instituted a new electronic medical record system that the rehab staff was unfamiliar with, and then criticized the staff for not having the patients' plan of care up to date. The policies and procedures regarding documentation were being carried out according to the "old" policy manual, which left the therapy staff members vulnerable when they had to defend themselves at staff meetings. The therapy staff members generally felt sabotaged, and the new administrative team perceived them as being less than competent with respect to documentation.

The importance of collaboration

Such situations do not make for the best patient care, nor do they create an environment that enhances recruitment and retention.

When you are ready to establish goals to enhance interdisciplinary or collaborative practice, begin with a process that causes staff members to take a step back and truly understand what collaborative practices are about. One way to initiate this process is to have the therapy staff, and all the professional departments, participate in a survey that asks questions such as the following:

- What does the term "collaborative practice" mean to you?

- Do you feel that by improving collaborative efforts we improve patient care?

- What are two things you can do to improve/enhance collaborative practice?

- What are two things other professionals can do to enhance collaborative efforts?

- Would you be interested in being part of a team that works with administration on a project targeted to improve collaborative practices in our organization?

You can use this survey to begin to educate staff members about collaboration by giving them a question that requires them to look at the literal definition of the term. For example:

> Which of the following terms are synonyms for collaboration?
> Joint, group effort, two-way, relationship, mutual, cooperation, shared, teamwork

This type of exercise reminds people that collaboration is more than cosigning standing orders or serving on the same committee.

Successful collaboration

Managers must lead by example to establish good relationships with coworkers. For instance, the physical therapy budget is being challenged, and the result is that some therapists will be required to administer specific passive range-of-motion exercises that previously had been administered by aides from the nursing department. Using collaborative practice, the managers of these two departments worked together before approaching their staff members.

When they were ready to present the change at the staff level, they continued the collaboration process by doing it at a joint staff meeting to show they were working as a team to identify the best approach to this challenge. This scenario reminds us that if managers work in collaboration with other managers, they can much more reasonably expect staff members to do so.

Collaboration is facility-wide

When therapists hear the word "collaboration," they often think of other rehab staff members, due to the frequency of the interaction of the various therapies. In contrast, when medical staff members hear the word, they often think of working well within their own peer group. Your first step toward improving collaboration may be simply to raise awareness among all employees that all departments and all employees must collaborate in order to provide effective and safe patient care.

Case study

Problem relationships

The new rehab manager had been warned about the physiatrist who had such a difficult personality that many therapists and nurses feared calling him for clarification on specific patient orders. When he stepped off the elevator, staff members often scattered. His behavior was widely known, and in all the years that he had been part of the medical staff, no one had confronted him about his behavior, not even the administrative team.

At the beginning of the therapy grand rounds on Monday morning, the new manager joined the therapy and nursing team to see how things were going, and she ran into the physical medicine and rehabilitation physician, who was also participating. She had not yet had the opportunity to meet him, and he caught her off guard. He immediately began a verbal harangue, listing the things "her staff did wrong on weekend coverage" and asking, "How could you allow this?"

This was the therapist's first management position, and she was unprepared for such an abrasive situation, particularly in front of her employees and other staff members. She began to cry and went to her office to hide from him. Her reaction took the physician by surprise, and he left the unit without saying a word. The next day, the new therapy manager received flowers from the physician—and an in-person apology. This led to a collaborative discussion between the new manager and the physician, in which he revealed that he did not realize how his behavior had been affecting others.

The conversation also brought to light some issues related to some legitimate patient care weekend coverage concerns the physician had, which he had been expressing for years but which were ignored due to the lack of relationship between him and administration.

Challenges of the healthcare environment

The healthcare environment throws many challenges at us as we try to enhance our teams and learn to work more effectively with other departments. These challenges include overworked and tired staff members, high-acuity patients and stressful decision-making environments, and administration's unwillingness to address unacceptable behaviors.

We cannot allow these challenges to be an excuse for not moving forward with collaborative practices. For some organizations, the biggest hurdle may be to get past the concept of "that's the way we've always done it around here."

When we approach the concerns related to lack of communication, teamwork, and mutual respect and goals, we know one thing for sure: Most people want what is in the best interest of the patient. When looking at collaborative practice issues, be sure to address patient safety and outcomes. No matter how many interdisciplinary committees you have, they are worth little if you are not improving patient outcomes. Your efforts in every area should always aim to do so.

Leadership's role

Regional rehabilitation hospitals, such as those designated by state regulatory bodies, continue to guide us, through their successes, in ensuring that leadership plays a direct role in encouraging and nurturing collaborative practices. By gauging effectiveness and by measuring patient outcomes, we can show with certainty the success of efforts directed at team-building and improving communication processes and systems.

Because improving collaboration is an ongoing process that will require leadership oversight and management, develop some working goals to help you manage your efforts in enhancing collaboration:

1. Assess therapy and medical staff perceptions of the current status of collaboration.

2. Ask the organization's leadership staff members about their perceptions of the status of collaboration in the organization. Include midlevel managers in this assessment.

3. Identify two successful collaborative efforts that have occurred in the past one or two years, and review the following:

- Why were they successful?

- Is the effort still in progress?

- Who or what was the motivating force for the success?

- Were patient outcomes related, and if so, how were they measured?

4. Obtain input from rehab, nursing, and medical staff members on their perception of the top three patient care concerns that need collaborative attention.

5. Compare these results with the responses from the leadership team.

After you have collected information:

- Share responses to survey questions at the next management meeting

- Develop a collaborative improvement team, and have top management appoint people who submitted targeted comments and suggestions on their surveys

- Involve staff members who are responsible for compliance with The Joint Commission or CARF standards and risk management in your improvement processes

- Actively involve newly hired therapists and nurses and physicians so that you have staff members with fresh perspectives, unhindered by a history of events at your organization

- Include the concept of collaborative practice in the orientation process

Why we work here

Amanda has been a physical therapist on the inpatient rehab facility unit for three years, and Jim, a former college classmate, is relocating to her neighborhood because of a family move and is looking for a new job. Amanda is located in a large city, so the competition among local hospitals, nursing homes, and therapy clinics for physical therapists is fierce, with recruitment efforts often focused solely on the amount of money offered in sign-on bonuses.

The rehab department manager where Amanda works has made it a department standard that all therapy staff members be involved in patient care practices, systems, and shared accountabilities. Amanda knows that she is part of something special, from the self-scheduling concept on the unit to the committee directed by one of the referring neurologists. Jim asks Amanda what the hospital is really like:

Jim: "Tell me the real story about what goes on in that unit. I met with your manager yesterday, and you know they all make things sound great."

Amanda: "No place is perfect. You learn what becomes really important once you have been out of school and working for a while. But I never thought I would sit on a committee with a neurologist who actually listened to my ideas about acute stroke patients. Everyone thinks these patients can just be transferred here after a day in acute, but I told him about some situations we had over here, and he really listened. Having to take weekend coverage once a month is not ideal, but I value this place—knowing that the docs here respect me and that my input counts for something means I'll look for growth and development opportunities here."

The importance of collaboration in recruitment and retention

This process must not be done only at the top level of the administration. Instead, it needs to be brought down to the individual department level, where you will see the benefit it brings to recruitment and retention. Creating an environment of mutual collaboration leads not only to improved patient outcomes, but also to a positive work experience.

One of the most important aspects of this scenario is that all parties involved realize that their work is making a difference. For example, the neurologist should receive feedback about the impact he or she is having on staff recruitment and retention. If you don't share this type of information on a regular basis, you can easily lose some of your best cheerleaders for collaborative practice.

Create collaborative relationships between therapists, nurses, medical staff members, and other departments

Here are the necessary steps to create and build a collaborative atmosphere.

1. **Do not tolerate unacceptable behavior.** Would you want to show up for work or come in to see a new rehab patient on a Sunday afternoon if you knew that the person with whom you had to collaborate exhibited behavior that you would not tolerate in your house? Whether it is foul language, a rude tone of voice, or negative comments about you or your team, the bottom line is that if you would not tolerate it at home, you should not tolerate it at work.

   At home, we put kids in timeout for antisocial behavior; at work, we use job descriptions and the mission/vision statement to hold people accountable. Develop and enforce policies and procedures that identify your definition of disruptive or unacceptable behaviors. Include strong language that reflects the organization's unwillingness to tolerate these behaviors and what the disciplinary process will be for those who elect not to change.

2. **Educate management/employees on appropriate communication methods and tools.** This process should begin on the first day of orientation, and continue on an annual basis as well as being referenced in the organization's Code of Conduct. Communication can be accomplished through e-mail newsletters with sample scenarios or through a written annual commitment, in which all staff members sign an agreement to use appropriate communication. Have the medical staff sign one, have it enlarged, and display it over the visitor entry.

3. **Leadership must demonstrate commitment to this process through their actions.** They can do so in many ways, such as by ensuring not only that collaborative committees meet, but also that participants are comfortable sharing their thoughts and concerns. Rapid response to disruptive behaviors is another example of leadership expressing their seriousness about it.

4. **Recognize that doctors and therapists have learned to communicate in different styles and methods.** Between 1995 and 2003, the primary cause of sentinel events was problems with communication, according to The Joint Commission.[1] Therapists and nurses are taught to gather data, relay it to the doctor, and include every detail in documentation. Physicians are taught to discover the problem and work out what needs to be done to fix it. How can you reconcile these methods of communication? Start with making the staff aware of the differences.

5. **Involve the staff-level therapists in teams and committees.** Typically, as the manager, you may not be in your department on a regular basis the entire time that your department is open. To measure patient and staff needs throughout the therapy day, however, we need to involve the people who are working during those times. Therefore, do not discourage staff involvement by only holding meetings at 8 a.m. Instead, vary meeting and committee times to give off-shift staff members an opportunity to participate actively.

6. **Identify success elsewhere and mimic it**. Find elsewhere the success you are seeking, study how it was accomplished, and then model your organization's method on it. In building collaborative practices, our best resources are ourselves—we must share our successes with one another. Recognized rehab facilities, such as those rated by peers, are great examples for us in this way as well, and any time spent on a field trip to see them in action is well worth it.

7. **Relate patient outcomes to collaborative initiatives.** It is one thing to feel a part of the process; it is another to actually see and work with the patient benefits related to it. Communicate data related to initiatives that involve collaborative practice agendas, and then educate staff members as to how this information translates into improved patient care.

8. **Building relationships requires patience.** Be patient with yourself, your staff, and the overall organization as you identify goals and work toward attaining them. Changing and improving the practice environment by incorporating more teamwork and cooperation across departments and among professionals takes time. It will be an

ongoing and continuous effort that does not have an end point. It is one of those projects that should not have a completion target date—if it ends, you lose an important motivator for therapists to stay with the organization.

The benefits of participating in collaborative systems that improve patient care

How many times have you heard staff members talk about wanting to be more empowered to do things differently? Yet sometimes when we ask for input or involvement, there is a rush for the door because no one wants to participate. Managers and leadership need to realize that what they see as active involvement may not be what staff members see as active involvement.

Therapists who feel they are actively involved in patient care processes and decisions are more satisfied with their jobs. Your challenge is to explore more ways for staff members to feel empowered and involved, but you first have to step back and learn what their perceptions really are. You can do so through informal discussions in small groups, at staff meetings, or through written surveys.

Here are some key questions to consider:

- If you could be empowered to do one thing around here, what would it be?

- Do you feel you need a policy or procedure in writing to validate all the things you are already empowered to do?

- What would motivate you to become more involved in patient issues related to your department?

- What is going on now in your environment that has turned you away from any desire to become more involved?

- Do you feel you are working in an environment where you can share your thoughts, concerns, ideas, or suggestions comfortably?

The responses to these questions will help you identify your next steps to motivate and encourage staff involvement.

People need to see results

All too often staff members go to meetings, collect data, and talk about issues, but never see any results. Thus, for staff members to feel involved, follow-through is imperative.

Shared governance has become popular in healthcare organizations because it allows staff members to contribute to decisions about issues and processes and then actually see the results of their involvement. For example, try changing clinical medical staff committees into joint practice committees with rehab staff included.

Daily collaboration

It's important to realize and appreciate that collaboration can occur spontaneously.[2] As leaders, we must point out to our staff the collaborative efforts that are in place every day.

Case study

A joint effort

An elderly man is about to be discharged with the walker he brought to the ambulatory care surgery center at the hospital. The nurse in charge notices the patient cannot ambulate safely with this walker and is concerned that he may fall. The nurse brings this issue to the attention of the physician, and together they discuss the options they could consider. The nurse calls physical therapy for their perspective, and a plan is developed for the patient to use a walker on wheels, the physician agrees, and the patient is discharged later that day with a new set of "wheels." Although this situation may sound like basic communication, it is a great example of interdisciplinary practice with collaborative effort among nursing, medical staff, and physical therapy.

Seamless teamwork

The rehab unit therapy manager is walking down the hallway and sees one of the referring neurosurgeons. They exchange greetings, and the rehab manager asks the surgeon if she has a minute to talk while she walks with her. The rehab manager shares a concern about a new acute protocol that affects spinal cord injury patients and explains how the protocol affected a patient in ICU yesterday. The surgeon agrees that this issue is a concern. She mentions that there is a spine trauma committee meeting that day and invites the rehab manager to attend and share her concerns and ideas for how to prevent the situation from occurring again.

Case study

Overcoming emotions

Collaboration is about relationships and, therefore, will involve emotions. At times, these emotions can become obstacles to the effectiveness of your efforts, which reminds us why objectivity is necessary to guide the changes in how physicians and therapists communicate, how patient care decisions are made, and how all employees are held accountable for disruptive behaviors. Consider professional burnout, differences in opinion from cultural perspectives, and the lack of negotiating skills many staff members may have. Identify leaders who are charged not only with the physical energy to lead change, but also with the emotional energy and integrity to do so. Provide training to staff on addressing aggressive and unacceptable behaviors.

References

1. *Competency Manager Advisor,* HCPro, Inc. (February 2005), p. 7.

2. Deborah B. Gardner, PhD, RN, CS. "Ten Lessons in Collaboration"; *www.nursingworld.org,* January 2005.

Professional development

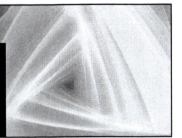

More than money

Studies remind us about the important role salary plays in recruitment and retention, but they also identify other important reasons why people accept or remain at a job. One item that always makes the list relates to professional development. It might be stated as training, education, or ongoing development, but regardless of what you call it, therapists want training and, for the most part, truly enjoy continuing education programs that meet their learning needs. They also want to be treated and respected as professionals and sometimes find themselves trapped between what they learn professionalism is versus what they think it should be.

What is professionalism?

Demonstrating professionalism

As in any situation, the manager needs to set an example of professionalism, and when it comes to professional development, staff members will watch to see what you do for your own personal training and growth. They watch what you wear and how you carry and present yourself to patients, medical staff, and administration.

Leading by example

Demonstrate your own professionalism in the following ways:

- At meetings or in other communications, reference something you learned from a class, self-study CD, or article you read. Let the staff know where the information came from.

"I was impressed by what I learned about verbally de-escalating angry patients and families in one of the sessions I attended at my conference last month. I brought copies of the handout

material to our meeting today so that I could share this information with you to get your insights to see whether it is an approach we should consider for our department."

- Post notices or place a note via e-mail or in the communication book when you are going to be away at a class.

  "I will be out of town with my cell phone off during class time while I attend the update on changes in Medicare documentation. When I return, I will fill you in on what the changes will mean for our documentation policies and procedures."

- Attend some classes with your staff, such as a CPR renewal course.

- Leave a copy of the brochure of a conference you will be attending, with the specific workshops you are scheduled for highlighted so that staff members can review them.

  If you are going back to college to obtain an advanced degree, talk about your course, the professors, and what you are learning. Consider posting a countdown calendar for staff members to see where you are in the program and what your timeline and goals are for completion.

- Demonstrate the importance of supporting your specialty organization by displaying posters, wearing a membership pin, or getting involved in state chapter efforts.

- Bring in your professional journal issues to share with the staff.

- Always follow the dress code policy. Look in the mirror before you leave for work, and ask yourself whether the patients and medical staff see from your physical appearance that you are an authority figure—and a professional one at that.

As you work toward implementing these practices, be careful not to set unrealistic expectations of staff members. They will not all run out and join their professional organizations, nor will they all read the conference brochure you posted, but they will all know that their manager is using current knowledge and skills to lead the patient care in their department. You are sending a strong message of professionalism, maturity, and accountability. These three elements related to professional development truly reflect its meaning and help us understand the enticing role it plays in therapy recruitment and retention.

What professionalism means to you and your staff

What does the word "professionalism" mean to you as the manager, and what does it mean to your staff and the prospective staff you interview? It can imply many things, such as being an expert or being trained/skilled in a specialty. It is your professionalism that is reflected when you elect to show up for work wearing clean white shoes, instead of the same sneakers you wore when you mowed the lawn. Relate your personal definition of professionalism to that of your staff.

The manager can gain this insight by talking with staff members and having them share their perceptions. Using group techniques, you can collect and share this information as part of a learning process at a staff meeting. Ask each staff member to write on a card two words or statements that define professionalism. Collect the cards, and using a grease board or flip chart, ask one staff member to read each response while another staff member writes them down for all to see. Refer to Figure 7.1 for a sample chart. While the staff members are writing down their comments, advise them that you have already written your definition of being professional and that you will share it with them after their cards are read and posted. Give the staff members an opportunity to discuss the responses from their peers, and then reveal your perception of being professional, which may look similar to Figure 7.2.

Figure 7.1	Being professional is . . .
• Being skilled at what you do	√ √ √ √
• Presenting yourself in an ethical manner	√ √
• Having current knowledge in your practice specialty	√ √ √ √ √ √
• Acting with respect toward your coworkers and patients	√ √ √
• Meeting the standards of what is expected of you	√
• Complying with rules and regulations of your profession	√ √ √ √ √ √
• Working together as a team	√ √

√ = for each person with a similar or like response

> ### Figure 7.2 | The manager's perception of being professional
>
> - Meeting the standards of your practice specialty
>
> - Behaving, dressing, and presenting yourself in an ethical and appropriate manner
>
> - Taking personal accountability for attendance and participation in educational events, staff meetings, and so on
>
> - Maintaining a current knowledge base of your practice specialty
>
> - Supporting your practice specialty national and state organizations and standards of practice

In the next exercise, ask staff members to write down one incident that has happened that they felt did not represent professional actions—and be careful to ensure that no one uses any names. Once again, collect and post these results, and open the floor for discussion. Doing so gives you and the staff an opportunity to discuss actual scenarios which you or the staff would not want to be representative of your profession. Here are examples that could be discussed:

- A COPD patient entered the facility for a therapy appointment through the wrong door and was met by a staff member taking a cigarette break.

- A therapist asks you to take care of entering a plan of care for her because she missed the training session on the new form and doesn't know how to enter the data online. She is whining and complaining about all the education the facility requires.

No one wants to work in an environment where these types of behaviors occur regularly. Therapists want to be surrounded by others who believe professionalism is important.

Maturity

How many times have you said to yourself: "I just wish some of these people would grow up"? Some therapy staff members may have similar thoughts about some of their coworkers. They want to be part of a team where maturity sets the pace for character development and decision-making. And as your staffing needs grow, you may find yourself in a position in which you are accepting more new therapists who for the first time are dealing with work responsibilities, let alone clinical responsibilities.

Making decisions about when to take a lunch break can seem minimal in how they affect others, yet in a rehab clinic, such decisions will affect patient and staff scheduling. It takes time and patience to help our new graduates grow and mature, and they deserve to receive help in the form of our demonstration of seasoned decisions and solid character that defines what being a professional is all about.

Accountability

Whatever you do, don't let staff members know that accountability and empowerment are the same thing—because if you do, many of them won't want to be empowered anymore. As managers, we hold ourselves accountable to ourselves, the staff, our patients, and the organization.

The professional therapist will want to be held accountable in the same manner and will be willing to do what it takes to show this level of responsibility. However, because there will always be staff members who feel that they do not have to be accountable to anyone except themselves, management must step forward and be the entity holding everyone to the same level of accountability.

Each time the manager takes steps to hold the staff accountable he or she sends important messages about professionalism. Staff members who are accountable and responsible will walk with heads held high, knowing that you respect their choices and that you see them as the professionals they are.

Accountability

Kimberly received a letter from the state board of occupational therapy stating that they had not received her renewal and that her license was due to expire that week. She realized that when she moved to a new apartment, she had neglected to send them her forwarding address. She took responsibility for this oversight, and she made time to drive the two hours to the office and pay the late fee to renew her license.

Jason is in the same situation, but he feels that the clinic should have a process in place to remind him. After all, he is busy with other things in his life. Are you going to hold Jason accountable? Will he be taken off the therapy schedule without pay as soon as his license is invalid? Your staff is watching to see what will be done and is proud when the organization takes steps to ensure that therapists hold themselves accountable to such issues related to professionalism.

Case study

Attending classes

Melinda had the same opportunities as the rest of the staff to select from one of four dates to attend a mandatory update educational session for the department. She did not attend any of them and did not let her manager know about any problems keeping her from doing so. The facility's policy states that staff members who do not attend cannot be placed on the time sheet without the manager's approval. Physical therapy is currently short-staffed and Melinda knows this, and she is currently signed up for weekend coverage. Are you going to take her off the schedule? Once again, the staff is watching you to see whether you will hold everyone accountable to the same level of responsibility.

Continuing education requirements

Your state board of speech–language pathology has enacted new standards regarding continuing education requirements, and you have posted some information, along with a Web site, for the staff to use to reference the specifics. Virginia is now in your office saying that she is angry that "you did not notify her" of these changes, and she doesn't remember getting any notification in the mail either. She was unable to renew her license because she did not have adequate continuing education validation to present with her renewal application. Are you going to put the accountability back in her lap?

Here's a sample script for how you could respond to Virginia: "Virginia, if you look at your current license, it has your name on it—not mine and not the facility's. That means you are personally accountable and responsible not only for knowing what the requirements are, but also for meeting them. It is unfortunate that you did not review the communication board two months ago when I posted the notice regarding this change."

Requirements for professional development

The education and training aspect of professionalism is driven from a variety of directions. Specific requirements may be set through various entities, such as The Joint Commission, CARF, Medicare, your state licensing board, your facility's policy, specialty standards, or other regulatory bodies. It is also a self-driven force, as people strive for professional development for reasons of personal fulfillment and challenge.

Encouraging education and training

Developing your therapy staff requires coaching from you, especially for new grads. Develop a resource list that staff members can use to access information about the requirements to obtain education, as well as information on where they can find the resources.

Figure 7.3 is an example of a resource list for rehab managers in an inpatient rehabilitation facility.

Figure 7.3 | **Sample professional development resources**

Organizations

American Medical Rehab Providers Association

American Hospital Association–Section for Long Term Care and Rehabilitation

Journals

Rehab Management: The Interdisciplinary Journal of Rehabilitation

PT Magazine

Books

Physical Therapy Management

(By Ronald W. Scott, PT, JD, EdD, LLM, MSBA, and Christopher L. Petrosino)

Web sites

www.aha.org

www.apta.org

www.asha.org

www.aota.org

www.amrpa.org

www.enw.org

Colleges and universities

Local college or university for courses and advanced training

School of Public Health

College of Business

Fulfilling the training and educational needs of therapists should be viewed from both a short-term and a long-term perspective. Therapists may need to acquire certain skills for the position they hold now, but it is important to incorporate education that gives them a focal point for some of their long-term goals, which may be three years from now.

Managers need not feel threatened by the therapist who is returning to school part time. Imagine a situation in which John, one of your physical therapists, is attending school part time to get his MBA. You may worry that you'll lose the best clinical person you have when John finishes school, but you have to remember the bigger picture. John may be moving on to other opportunities when he completes his goals, but look at the benefit that you, the staff, and the patients are gaining while he is there for two more years. For now, John is:

- A role model and mentor for the staff

- A therapist with advanced assessment skills who can help his peers improve their own assessment skills

- A staff member with a higher sense of responsibility, both clinically and ethically

- A therapist who, while in business school, will focus on identifying particular clinical concerns that will improve patient outcomes

Another way to approach the situation is from the professional development perspective by asking whether there is a need in the department that John can fill when he completes his training. Have you been thinking of hiring an outpatient manager with business expertise, which is necessary to compete in the outpatient rehab setting? Part of our job as managers is to help staff members develop their professional growth by guiding them in career choices.

Highlight your staff's successes

John will always remember the manager who supported him while he was in school, and he will take particular pride in the organization that backed his decision with a flexible schedule. This is an amazing recruitment and retention opportunity and an example of where you can use your bragging rights to aid in recruitment and retention efforts. Shout John's successes from the rooftops by:

- Posting on the hospital Web site (with his permission) a photo of John with "his story," describing his career choice and how he is making it happen

- Placing a photo of you and John in the local community newspaper when he completes his MBA program, and including comments about his career path and how the organization supported him

- Using the same photos and stories in your therapy recruitment ads or brochures

You should be very proud of what John has accomplished and that you are part of an organization that supports this type of professional development.

Offer access to continuing education

Encourage professional development by providing programs such as on-site education. Your time and financial investment in such programs will come right back to you in recruitment and retention—managers with reputations of supporting continuing education are the ones whose vacancies fill quickly. When staff members are supported and encouraged to attend educational offerings, it sends a message that the organization values them and their capabilities.

Therapists feel appreciated when their organization goes a step further and sends them off-site to national conferences. When you look at the overall costs for doing so compared to the cost of recruiting and orienting another therapist, the numbers speak for themselves.

Your role in shaping future careers

Now that you realize that professional development involves more than ensuring that staff members renew their CPR cards, position yourself with information that helps you look at your staff members' individual career choices and paths. Some will prefer to stay at their current level, but five years from now, that may change. You never know when the opportunity you give a therapist will affect the development of a peer. Using tools such as the ones in Figure 7.4 and Figure 7.5 can help both you and the new grad or experienced therapist plan for current and future skills and educational needs. Figure 7.6 can be customized to set long-term goals.

Figure 7.4 | Rehabilitation department—sample professional development

New-graduate therapist

Employee name:

Date of hire:

Date of graduation from PT/OT/SLP school:

Date of successful completion of:
1. State licensing exam
2. National certification

Education (Course or training)	Target date	Resource	Date completed/comments
Transitioning from student to professional	30 days of hire	In-house class	
Medicare compliance: rehab risk area training	30 days of hire	In-house class	
Documentation to the electronic medical record	15 days of hire	Facility intranet self-paced course	
CPR		Community college	

Figure 7.5 | Rehabilitation department—sample professional development

Experienced therapist

Employee name:

Date of hire:

Practice specialty: PT/OT/SLP/Other

Current certifications:

Professional development plan for _____ (insert year):

Education	Target date	Resource	Date completed/comments
NDT course		Off-site clinical course	
Progressing to a supervisory position		In-house training	
CPR recertification		Community college	

Additional professional development:
1. Has requested to be considered for future supervisory openings
2. Presented a class for the hospital community education program on "Falls prevention within the home"

Notes:
This employee has expressed an interest in going back to school to begin courses in the MPH program at the College of Medicine with assistance from the tuition reimbursement program.

Figure 7.6 | Rehabilitation department—sample career path

Today's date:

Name:

Current position:

Department/section:

	1 year	2 years	3–5 years	Comments
Staff therapist				
Rehab supervisor	√			Will be scheduled for upcoming in-house courses and webinars
Returning to school		√		MPH program part time
Advancing to a hospital (rehab) management position			√	

Tie professional development into recruitment and retention

As you continue to develop what you offer therapy staff members in terms of their professional growth, always consider how you can tie these efforts into recruitment and retention:

- Place a photo and story in the local newspaper about the therapists who recently completed their specialty certifications

- Use your Web site to spotlight quotes from new grads and new hires about how wonderful your orientation process is and how they are elated with the ongoing education offered on-site at no cost

- Work with a community newspaper to have therapists involved in writing a monthly column related to a timely health issue, such as preventing slips and falls in the home

Employees want professional development

The Society for Human Resource Management addressed the issue of staff turnover in a survey that examined what people were really looking for in their jobs and careers. The second biggest reason they would begin searching for a new job was dissatisfaction with potential career development. The third reason was readiness for a new experience. This information highlights the importance of your professional development efforts.

When focusing on the retention side of professional development, ask yourself these questions:

- What processes are in place to have staff members provide some of the training themselves?

- What opportunities are there for staff members to cross-train so that they can decide whether they want to pursue other specialties or interests in the organization?

- When was the last time you gave staff members an opportunity to express what their other interests are and how they see themselves incorporating them into their job?

- How often is the staff given an opportunity to participate in committees or teams?

- Are staff members able to use some of their talents, skills, and knowledge at occasions outside the building, such as at a health fair or a senior citizen blood pressure screening?

Focusing on what really matters

Troy is about to graduate from physical therapy school. He has worked as a physical therapy tech for two years, and he knows that this exposure has increased his comfort level when working with patients. As he excitedly starts setting up job interviews, he is overwhelmed by all the offers for hourly salary rates, sign-on bonuses, and other tempting incentives. However, many of the therapists he worked with previously had given him advice about what to look for in his first job, and they suggested that he focus on what the organizations offered in terms of continuing education and work environment.

After two years of working for little more than minimum wage, Troy is initially drawn by the glitter of the salary. However, those experienced therapists had a great effect on him, and he eventually opts for a position with less pay but with an excellent program for new-graduate orientation and a department manager who is overtly committed to ongoing training for the staff. As he settles into his new role, he hears feedback from his former schoolmates and realizes that he has made the best decision for his professional development. His schoolmates share stories of their experiences, ranging from one who receives little new-graduate support to one who is expected to start as the only therapist in the skilled nursing unit the next month and who is so overwhelmed by this responsibility that he is looking for a new job already.

Professional development should begin from day one after graduation and be an ongoing process throughout a therapist's career. New grads need some dedicated time and guidance to transition in their roles. Facilities with these programs are more enticing to new therapists.

Beverly L. Kaye and Sharon Jordan-Evans write that, "Our research shows that more than any other single factor, people stay in an organization because of opportunities to stretch, grow and learn."[1] Relating this research to professionalism is vital to reducing employee turnover and hiring the best for the team.

From the time you make a decision to hire or recruit an individual therapist, think about how you will encourage him or her regarding career goals, education, and training. Your leadership will drive his or her professional development and, therefore, the standards of the department. (See Figure 7.7 for a professional development pyramid.)

Figure 7.7 | Professional development pyramid

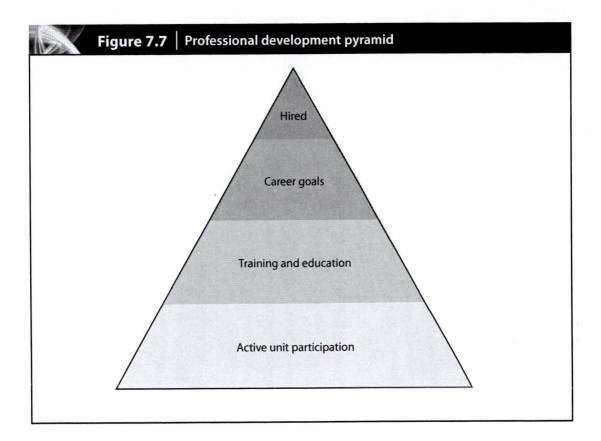

Quality patient care will result from your staff's professional development, and patients will see their caregivers' commitment to delivering the very best. Staff members will feel good about being part of a team they know is qualified and competent to meet the needs of their patients. Never forget the importance of your role as you recruit, interview, and work to keep the staff as professional as you already have.

References

1. Beverly L. Kaye and Sharon Jordan-Evans. *Love 'Em or Lose 'Em: Getting Good People to Stay* (San Francisco: Berrett-Koehler Publishers, 1999).

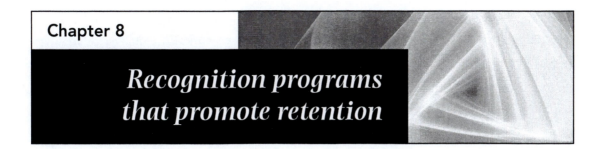

Chapter 8

Recognition programs that promote retention

The importance of recognition and reward programs

Recognizing and rewarding employees are integral components of any retention program. Work in healthcare organizations is laborious and stressful, and most therapists choose their career because of an inherent desire to make a difference in people's lives. Recognition of their contributions to quality patient care and peer relations affirms that they are succeeding in making a positive difference.

Most healthcare employees are motivated by a passion for caring for others—both patients and colleagues. For a majority of therapists, recognition and reward for exceptional contributions to patients and colleagues demonstrate appreciation, value, and caring by peers, managers, administration, and the healthcare organization.

Principles of recognition and reward programs

Consider several principles as you develop recognition and reward programs and activities. There's nothing worse than thinking you have a thoughtful, exciting new way to recognize staff members, only to realize that your employees did not appreciate the effort at all.

Be genuine in all of your activities, and make recognition personal

You must be sincere and genuine in any recognition or reward action. Staff members quickly realize whether your words or actions are appropriate for the occasion. Your thoughts do not have to be inspired, but they must be inspiring. It can be as simple as "I appreciate what you do," or "You are an important part of our healthcare team." Keep thank you notes available at all times, and make a goal of writing at least five every few weeks. Keep them simple and personal. Most people have experience working with a supervisor who provides a pat on the back and positive comments only when he or she wants you to work an extra shift—as the supervisor begins to commend the employee on his or her work, the employee is already thinking of reasons why he or she can't work on the weekend. The purpose of recognition and rewards is to sincerely thank someone for something already given, not to warm him or her up for something you want.

Award recognition and rewards fairly and equitably

A cardinal rule of healthcare is to "do no harm," and the same holds true for recognition and rewards. Your goal is to demonstrate appreciation for a job well done, but you don't want to alienate certain groups of employees. For example, although it's great to recognize occupational therapists during National Occupational Therapy Week, you'll want to make sure you have an opportunity to recognize social workers, physicians, and housekeeping staff as well during their special weeks. Make sure you have a fair and equitable process for selecting recipients for individual recognition. Develop criteria for each award that is given. If you serve as the master of ceremonies for an award event, never say, "The winner is . . .," but rather "The award goes to . . ." Also, describe the specific behavior that was observed and that warranted the recipient receiving the award.

Ask staff members how they would like to be recognized

You might form a Recognition and Reward Task Force to survey or hold a brainstorming session to determine ways in which staff members prefer to be recognized.

Some people prefer death to speaking in front of a group, so always ask staff members whether they would like a few moments to speak. If you plan to put together a bulletin board and include staff photos, ask them how they feel about it. Some staff members prefer no public recognition, but they may really like to be recognized in a private manner, such as with a letter or a certificate. Others love to be recognized publicly. Therefore, know which staff members prefer which types of recognition.

Case study

Inappropriate form of recognition

Judy was a quiet, reserved occupational therapy assistant who had performed excellent care for several years and was rewarded with an Excellent Patient Care Award. As she received the award in front of the group, she was asked to say a few words. It was immediately obvious that she had no idea she would be asked to speak and was surprised and embarrassed in front of the group.

Individualize recognition activities

Know your employees' life interests and priorities, and look for a great recognition or reward action that matches those interests. If an employee is an avid golfer, her reward might be a dozen of her favorite golf balls or a round of golf at a local course. For someone who knits or crochets, it might be the latest wool, or scarf pattern. The most effective actions match the employee's life interests and priorities.

Case study

Personal touch

Diane was the organization's therapy recruiter who consistently exceeded recruitment goals and was being recognized for the fourth year in a row for her exceptional recruiting. The director of the human resources department asked her to attend the annual awards luncheon to accept the beautiful plaque that the healthcare system usually provided. As the director delivered the award, Diane remarked, "Thank you, but to be honest, I have a wall full of these awards."

Diane continued to excel, and in year five, she once again won the award. The director had learned an important lesson, and she knew the love of Diane's life was her three-year-old Beagle named Watson. She secretly arranged for a colleague who kept Watson when Diane was out of town to bring Watson to a professional photographer to have photo taken. At the luncheon, as Diane walked to the front of the room, the director said, "We hope you know how much we love what you do for us," as she unveiled the beautiful framed photo of Watson. Diane was teary-eyed, and for the first time in a long time, she was speechless.

Make recognition and reward a part of your work culture

Make formal and informal recognition and reward a usual and customary part of your everyday work life. Establish formal recognition programs such as Employee of the Month and Employee of the Year. Encourage staff members to recognize positive behaviors in colleagues on a daily basis. Make recognition a part of your staff meetings.

Make formal recognition events thoughtful and majestic

If you already have a nice Employee of the Month or Employee of the Year event and have held it for several years, you must make the event fresh and engaging each year. You do not need to increase your cost for the event, but you do need to integrate new thoughts and ideas. For example, change the theme or change the venue. You must romance your staff: The ceremony must be thoughtful, it must be meaningful, and it must include something unexpected.

Even though you provide an excellent luncheon and special memento to celebrate National Rehab Week, it won't be long before attendees begin to say, "It's the same thing we've been doing for the past three years." Mix it up. You might do a casual luncheon one year and a formal dinner the next. When recognizing employees of the year, you might use an "Evening of the Stars" theme. One recruiter used an "Oscar Night" theme and hired an actor who performed as a live Oscar statue.

Examples from practice

A large public hospital (with an inpatient rehab unit, an acute care clinic, a therapy burn unit, and multiple rehab outpatient clinics) recommends the following examples of formal and informal recognition and reward activities and peer recognition activities that have been used over the years and whose proven practices can be adapted for any organization.

Formal recognition and rewards

- Create a formal recognition committee to nominate and submit applications to recognize staff members. Committee membership consists of rehab staff members who represent all service lines and clinics. Staff members are chosen for clinic as well as hospitalwide recognitions.

- Provide a recognition breakfast or lunch for those who work to advance their skills to higher certification or license levels; for example, an occupational therapy assistant completing requirements to become an occupational therapist.

- Recognize staff members who have perfect attendance on a quarterly basis.

- Award an "Employee of the Month Rehab Spirit Award," and make each recipient eligible for an annual "Spirit" prize. Awardees' names are placed into a drawing for a vacation trip, conference attendance fees, or some other meaningful prize. Patients as well as staff members can nominate individuals for this award.

- Hand out "Staff Awards" at each staff meeting for someone who has gone "above and beyond" and give a small gift, such as a Starbucks gift card.

Informal recognition and rewards

- Recognize a staff member for a job well done in front of other staff members on a daily basis.

- Hand out movie tickets for two when someone needs encouragement, and include a note that says "Look at the big picture and know you are appreciated."

- Display banners that list the years of service for all staff members. Provide a tally to demonstrate the total years of service on a unit.

- Begin each staff meeting with recognition of staff members mentioned on patient satisfaction surveys or thank you cards from patients.

- Develop an "Extra Mile Award" for extraordinary accomplishments made outside your staff members' normal jobs.

- Give individual staff members their own day. Recognize special people, achievements, or actions by declaring a work date as their day. Announce that next Tuesday is "Chris Smith Day," and ask all the staff members to say or do something to contribute to the celebration.

- Recognize good performers by addressing the problems of poor performers. Letting others get away with subpar behavior is a slap in the face to the majority of those who carry their share of the load—and more.

- Frequently point out what a great team you have to upper management and administration.

- Send pizza with a "thanks for all you do" note when things are hectic in a clinic or on a unit.

- Appear in the clinic or on the unit with all the fixings to host an ice cream social.

Encourage peer recognition

Consider the following tactics for encouraging peer recognition:

- Place a journal on each unit, and dedicate it to staff members at the beginning of the year for them to record when coworkers do something nice or above and beyond expectations, so they can share each other's accomplishments.

- Encourage staff members to e-mail you with good things about each other, and read the notes in staff meetings.

- Develop recognition stickers and make them available for staff members to give to each other when they do something good. For example, a sticker might read, "I made a difference today!"

- Encourage the staff to provide a verbal thank you to coworkers on a daily basis.

- Supply a "recognition box" with cards, sticky notes, happy-face stickers, and other supplies, and place it in a common area. Encourage people to use material from the box frequently to acknowledge coworkers' good performance. Remember that you set the example.

A pat on the back or other acknowledgment provides positive reinforcement. In the busy, hectic, stressful days of providing quality healthcare, such an acknowledgment can reaffirm to staff members that they are making a difference in peoples' lives. Make recognition and rewards a part of your everyday work culture. Make it genuine. Make it personal. Make it meaningful.

Performance reviews are vital to retention

A waste of time

Annie has been a physical therapist in the acute care hospital at her healthcare organization for 13 years, and her annual review is coming up next week. The evaluation process at her facility offers no challenges for a physical therapist with Annie's experience, as her salary has been capped and she views the evaluation process as a waste of her time. A different perspective is provided by her boyfriend, Peter, who has been a physical therapist for five years at a different hospital. Since Peter's new rehab manager, Sandra, started two years ago, employees have actually become excited about preparing for their annual reviews, and turnover has decreased.

Case study

Why performance reviews matter

Annie's lack of an effective performance review may contribute to her lack of commitment toward her manager and her facility. If employees are not committed, they're likely to look for more attractive options elsewhere. This is one reason why effective performance reviews are vital retention tools that should become part of your ongoing retention efforts.

To better understand the importance of the relationship between performance review and staff retention, consider the preceding scenarios. What is Peter's manager doing that has staff members viewing their annual reviews positively? Reflect for a few minutes on comments often heard from therapists when asked about performance reviews or annual evaluations:

- "The only purpose of my annual review is to determine what percentage salary increase I get. For me, the 2.5% difference isn't worth the time of the review."

- "What performance are they reviewing? Everyone knows it doesn't matter how many inservices you skip or how rude you are—those people are still here, aren't they?"

Annie may still be at her job despite her attitude about the annual review, but the important question is whether her performance is up to par. You can hang on to all the employees you want, but if they are poor performers, would you want to be a part of that team?

Evaluate your programs

An effective retention program needs to incorporate performance reviews that accomplish something and that both management and staff can trust. Before you begin a program or revitalize your existing one, consider that an effective program should clearly identify employees' strengths and weaknesses and guide them in goal setting. It also should support the manager's efforts.

Keep ongoing records

Think back to your experiences as a new manager, when you reviewed previous evaluations of staff. It's likely that, as you were reading some of them, you were thinking, "Someone must have put the wrong name on this one because there is no way Jeremy does all these things. I may have been here for only three months, but I know he is rarely on time." Remember these enlightening moments the next time you are unsure whether to document something on an employee's annual review. The process is not just for the employee—it is also for the manager, the organization, and any new manager that may step into that role unexpectedly.

Four steps to effective performance reviews

Follow these steps when reviewing how you currently work with staff members at the time of their annual review or evaluation.

Step 1: Set the stage

Helping the employee feel prepared is as important as getting yourself ready, and you can accomplish this goal in numerous ways.

For example, send a letter or e-mail to employees that confirms the date and time of the review. Outline any material they are required to bring with them. Ask them to review a copy of their job description, and plan to discuss it. Remind them about where they can find this (such as in the department policy manual; do not include a copy of it with the letter). You may consider having them present five charts that demonstrate evidence of documentation standards or, possibly, a list of the continuing education activities in which they have participated during the past year.

Encourage them to bring copies of letters from coworkers or patients that recognize their efforts as a way to demonstrate the importance of their role to the department and the organization. Because coaching the employee to set goals is such an important aspect of this annual review, take the opportunity in your letter to include a worksheet to help guide the employee in setting these goals (see Figure 8.1).

Figure 8.1 | Goals worksheet

Name: _____

Job title: _____

Today's date: _____

Short-term goals for the coming year

In the next year, I would like to do the following:

Upgrade my clinical skills in the following areas:

_____

Take continuing education classes in the following areas:

_____

Work on the following projects:

_____

Long-term goals

In the next 3–5 years I would like to do the following:

Have completed:

_____

Make these changes in my career:

_____

Have accomplished: _____

Step 2: Prepare for the review

Remember, the annual review should not be the first time employees hear negative or positive comments regarding their performance. They should be able to walk into the meeting with no surprises thrown at them. You should be prepared with the following:

- Documentation to support your discussion of both positive and negative comments. Include copies of letters or notes from the employee's peer group, evidence of time sheets with tardy dates if attendance is an issue, or incident reports from multiple occurrences of similar events.

- A clear perspective on what you want to communicate about the employee's work performance.

- How you see the employee getting more involved in patient outcomes.

- A plan that includes clear expectations and timelines for changes in unacceptable behavior.

Figure 8.2 | Manager resources for annual review process

- Related to the employee:
    - Employee self-evaluation including future goals
    - Employee's current job description
    - Previous year's evaluation for comparison and reference
    - E-mails or letters complimenting the employee
    - Records of committee involvement
    - Pertinent attendance records (departmental meetings, trainings, overall attendance)
    - Salary history/information
    - Results of quality assurance activities, chart audits, productivity
    - Other individual statistical summaries
- Related to the organization:
    - Employee handbook
    - Organization Mission Statement and Code of Conduct
    - Department goals
    - Applicable policies and procedures

[Copies of patient charts that express good documentation skills]

Motivate

Byron: I don't care about the goals thing. Just put down that I'll renew my required certifications again: They're both due this year for recertification. Not everyone wants to go get a DPT, you know.

Manager: You are right about that—I have no aspirations to get a DPT either. But that doesn't mean I don't have any goals. For example, on my performance review, I put down that one of my goals was to take a healthcare finance course to better understand the budget process, maybe even explore taking some MBA courses. Setting goals isn't always about taking a class or achieving certification. It is about where you see yourself heading over the next year or two while you are in this job. So, with that in mind, where do you see yourself over the next year?

Byron: I do think about the time I am away from my kids and wish I could be there to do more things with them. I wish I wasn't gone so much—I miss lots of their school stuff that I wanted to be a part of now that they are a little older.

Manager: I appreciate your sharing that with me because it will help us set your goals for next year. You mentioned that you wanted more time for the kids' school activities, so have you thought about working the early schedule from 6 a.m.– 1:30 p.m. so that you would be home when the kids get out of school? You could try it for six months, and at the end of the six months you can decide whether you want to do that on a regular basis. With the great feedback I get on your team-leading skills, you would be perfect for lead physical therapist in the acute care clinic.

Byron: I didn't know that I could do that on a temporary basis. Can I sign up for that now?

- Resource tools to validate your comments or plan of action (see Figure 8.2).

Step 3: Focus on the goals

This conversation has allowed the manager to identify the catalyst that will help Byron meet a personal need, which will thereby enhance his professional performance. At the same time, the manager may gain an effective leader for the weekend team. By working together to set goals, the manager sets out on a communication path to try to find what inspires and motivates the employee. Remember, employees who are happy and fulfilled with their home status reflect similar characteristics at work.

Goal-setting has to be perceived by the employee as more than filling in the blanks on a form. If the manager minimizes the goals, the employee will never get the connection between job performance and having aspirations or ambition to do more.

When employees know that their manager supports their goals and are asked to be a part of the solution for challenges in the department, they become team players. This feeling leads to commitment, which is your retention motivator. The real test for the manager is to find a process that allows you to incorporate the annual review into daily practice. Gather information throughout the year. Make small notes on staff performance, send e-mails to staff, talk to people at change of shift, and stop waiting for the annual performance review to be the one time when employees hear that they are doing a good job. Time spent with staff both on a formal and an informal basis provides the employee and the manager with an opportunity to look at performance issues more frequently.

Step 4: Have the employee feel he or she is a part of the change process for improvement

Prepare key questions that help prompt effective communication between the manager and the therapist. Consider providing the employee with this list of questions, along with the letter you send confirming his or her appointment for the review:

- If you had the power to change just one thing about this department, what would it be?

- Is there anything you have accomplished over the past year of which I am not aware that you would like to share with me?

- You are such an asset to this department and I appreciate all of your efforts and would like to know what motivates you to come to work every day.

- Where do you see our department heading in light of the recent issues and challenges we discussed at our last staff meeting?

- What can I, or our facility, do to help you do your job more effectively?

The role of rehab administration in recruitment and retention

A vast portion of the retention effort falls on the shoulders of the therapy managers. In today's world, midlevel managers are seeing their position shift to that of one comprising of recruitment and retention. Where does this leave rehab administration in relation to this vital piece of patient care?

Without specific guidelines and goals, the hospital or rehab administrator may be completely out of the loop until there is a crisis, such as a large turnover, or worse, a huge vacancy issue.

Become involved

To play an effective role in the recruitment and retention of therapists in your organization, consider these necessary functions of administration.

Leadership development: Ongoing leadership development for the midlevel manager is critical to the success you will have in retaining the therapy managers that work with you.

Direct involvement: Become directly involved in various aspects of recruitment and retention. Have monthly data forwarded to you regarding turnover, overtime, and agency staffing. Have exit interview forms from therapists copied for your review and follow-up. Discuss the recruitment and retention status of your staff at your regular manager meetings.

Visibility: Make yourself visible to the new hires. Introduce yourself at orientation. Once a month, meet with a newly hired therapist for coffee to get his or her perspective on the hiring process, orientation process, and job satisfaction.

Support: Support the orientation process. Allocate and support necessary funds for appropriate and productive orientation programs. Implement indicators for a quality review process of the orientation program. Have this data shared with all therapy supervisors and managers and set goals for improvements.

Listen: Approach some of the seasoned therapy staff members and ask them what keeps them there. Ask what they would like to see the organization implement to help retention efforts.

Therapy staff members want to feel a connection to key rehab administrative staff members, partly for professional reasons but also because they want you to know what a great job they are doing. Making time for them leaves a perception that you want to be aware of issues. Go to a department where a staff member has recently attained specialty certification, and have a picture taken with that person for the local community newspaper or facility Web site. Having pride in your profession not only provides a model for what we want to see in rehab staff members, but also leaves them with a feeling of self-worth that motivates them to stay.

Establishing an academic pipeline

Schools and programs geared toward the careers of allied health professionals provide the renewable resources you count on from year to year. Therefore, it's in the best interest of any healthcare organization to develop partnerships with these schools and programs to assist in student recruitment, student retention, faculty recruitment, faculty retention, clinical and classroom space, and even funding.

Recruit into the health professions

For many years, hospitals and healthcare employers have focused recruitment efforts only on therapy training schools, which cater to a group of people who have already decided to enter the healthcare profession. But if you focus on people before they reach that point, you can actively recruit people into the healthcare profession and expand your pool of potential employees.

Consider recruiting people into the health profession as a long-term strategy. Target youth, second-career individuals, older workers, and displaced workers. Provide opportunities for members of each of these groups to gain insight into the challenges and rewards of healthcare careers. You might hold career fairs, volunteer programs, shadow programs, or even summer healthcare career camps.

High Point (NC) Regional Health System provides a "Promoting Advancement for Teens in Healthcare" (PATH) Program. The PATH Program is a student volunteer experience that selects 60 high school students to volunteer for 50 hours in the summer. The program is directed by hospital volunteer services, and each student gets to experience many aspects of care, as well as being required to attend classes on customer service, health and wellness, and healthcare careers.

Highlight the variety and potential of healthcare careers

People choose a career in healthcare because they want to "help people" or "make a difference in people's lives." Share your own story about how you, as a healthcare professional, have achieved positive patient outcomes. Develop a two-minute personal experience story that describes how a patient who was experiencing several healthcare challenges achieves a positive outcome.

Develop several such stories to use for different occasions. For example, have different ones to share with middle or high school students and another for second-career or displaced workers. For the latter groups, you could share a story of career growth and satisfaction, such as how an employee began working as a therapy tech, and then through encouragement, financial assistance, and personal support is now working as a physical therapist in your organization.

Young people have several misperceptions about healthcare careers. As you develop stories, materials, or presentations for youth, highlight the following areas to challenge their preconceptions and to illustrate how therapy is an interesting, challenging, and diverse career.

We need smart people in healthcare

The fields of rehab present as an intellectually challenging career, but many youth do not think you need to be smart to become a therapist. The general perception is that other healthcare professionals take orders from physicians and that it does not require an intelligent person to carry out physicians' orders. Therefore, when you talk with young people, let them know that therapists must keep up with the latest clinical knowledge and that learning will be a life-long endeavor.

We need decision-makers in therapy

Some young people may believe that therapists are not autonomous professionals. Once again, the perception is that healthcare professionals carry out physicians' orders. Therefore, talk with youth about how a therapist is a collaborative member of the healthcare team and is responsible and accountable for the delivery of quality care. Help them understand that rehab managers are responsible for multimillion-dollar budgets and that, many times, it's the therapist who recognizes different interventions are needed to enhance patient outcomes. Help them understand that therapists make decisions that affect patient outcomes each moment of the day.

There is a lifetime of variety in rehab

Young people may assume that all therapists work in hospitals. Although many do, let them know about the numerous other employment settings and environments, such as nursing homes, rehab centers, outpatient clinics, schools, the military, cruise ships, or even with professional sports teams.

Let them know that therapists work with a variety of patients, from newborns to older adults. Also talk about the variety of specialties, including orthopedics, pediatrics, women's care, rehabilitation, burn care, neonatal intensive care, and sports medicine, just to name a few. If you grow tired of working in one area, with some retooling and development of additional skills you can transfer your skills to a different work setting or specialty.

Health careers offer opportunities for career progression

Many young people think that all you will ever do in therapy is direct patient care. First, let them know that you can progress your career within clinical care. Many hospitals and clinics offer career advancement programs that allow you to advance in pay and responsibility based upon work experience, formal education, and certification. Talk about the roles of management, education, and research.

Look at your organization's Web site

Most healthcare home pages focus on recruiting patients. Consider also placing a "Learn more about healthcare careers" button on your home page. If you have an "Employee of the Month" program, highlight the recipients, include photos, and describe their work responsibilities. Send an e-mail to local career exploration teachers in middle schools so that they can explore your numerous careers. Include other activities that demonstrate the rewards and challenges of healthcare careers.

Practical strategies for educating young people about allied healthcare careers

Newspapers in Education program

Most local newspapers provide the Newspapers in Education program. They contact teachers of career exploration courses and ask whether they would like to receive the paper at no charge to improve reading skills and to share career opportunities available in the local community. The newspaper then sells sponsorship space for career pages to local employers. Consider developing a page for this program on careers that you know will be in long-term demand. For example, you might do a full page that just generally focuses on therapy career opportunities. Or if you feel that students need a better explanation of the different roles in therapy, you might sponsor a page each on physical therapy, occupational therapy, speech–language pathology, physical therapy assistant, and occupational therapy assistant.

Speaker's bureau

You may already have a speaker's bureau of healthcare professionals who provide health prevention education to the public. If you do, expand it to include employees who have stellar work experiences with your organization and are willing to improve their speaking skills. Include representatives from housekeeping, the business office, the human resources department, nursing, respiratory therapy, and so on. Develop a public speaking course to help them develop their success stories and to articulate to the public what they love about their careers. Look for opportunities to speak to community groups of youth, displaced workers, individuals considering second careers, and older workers.

Host or lead a youth group

Encourage some of your employees to host a youth group that is interested in learning more about healthcare careers. The YWCA and YMCA host several youth groups that focus on career exploration. Some communities have career explorer clubs, and both the Girl Scouts and Boy Scouts of America include badge and patch programs that focus on career exploration.

Coloring pages, puzzles, and textbook covers

Look for opportunities to increase youth awareness of healthcare careers. For example, you can develop and place coloring pages on your Web site that depict careers in your organization, and then hold a coloring contest for National Rehab Week or some other celebration.

Word puzzles focusing on medical terminology or healthcare careers are another strategy. You can place them on your Web site, or distribute them to your physicians for placement in their office waiting areas. Develop a variety of activities, and place your organization's logo on each one.

Encourage the staff to get involved in community organizations

Most healthcare organizations encourage staff members to provide community service, and often the staff members choose to be involved in health prevention, fundraisers, and other health-related activities. Educational systems play a major role in exposing youth to career choices, so encourage some of your staff to participate in the following roles:

- President or member of the Parent Teacher Association in an elementary or middle school

- Member of the local board of education for the public school system

- Member of a board of advisors for local private schools

- Health Occupations Students of America advisor or healthcare career advisor in a local high school

- Member of a school of allied health program advisory committee

Develop relationships with schools of allied health

Take a look at your recent new graduates, and analyze where they are coming from and the schools they attended. You may find that most of the programs are in your state, but you also may learn that you hire graduates from programs that are not in your immediate hiring region.

Make a list of the allied health programs, and then determine where you have developed working relationships. Discuss with a recruiter or colleagues to make sure you have an organizational liaison that works closely with all of these programs to develop and maintain collaborative relationships. Designate someone in your agency to meet with the deans and directors at least once per year to discuss clinical rotations, student space needs, faculty orientation needs, and evaluations on student learning experiences. Some larger organizations are establishing full-time positions to work directly with the schools to arrange clinical rotations, faculty orientation, and so on.

Community meetings

Another strategy for coordinating student experiences and working together to address demand for healthcare professionals is to hold healthcare community meetings. For example, in Winston-Salem, NC, there is a Winston-Salem Healthcare Roundtable. The Chamber of Commerce hosts the meeting because it felt strongly that successful business and commerce depend upon the health and welfare of the area's citizens. Members of the Roundtable include local schools of nursing, hospitals, long-term care facilities, home health and hospice agencies, public school health occupations programs, and career awareness representatives.

Work with the schools

Develop working relationships with schools and educational programs by keeping faculty informed of what's going on in your facility. Send them copies of your organizational newsletter. Inform your staff about when and where student clinical experiences will be held.

Incorporate faculty into your workplace. Offer joint faculty-clinical appointments, or part-time employment opportunities. Use faculty to teach some of your continuing education programs. Use local faculty with research expertise to develop clinical research studies and opportunities.

Establish quality standards for great clinical experiences for your students. The rehab manager should welcome students in their first clinical rotation, inquire about how the experience can be improved, and provide follow-up within a week. Emphasize your facility's commitment to providing quality care and a quality learning experience. Ask for input on how you and your staff can help with and improve their experience. Inform them on how you will implement their suggestions. Keep them up to date on your progress.

Establish relationships with students

It is important to develop relationships with allied health students before they graduate. Hold open houses and career fairs to share information about working in your organization and to begin developing relationships with the students. Visit schools, and provide pizza for student-sponsored events throughout the year. Advertise in college-related publications or student association magazines or newsletters. Host a senior reception two or three months prior to graduation.

Maintain data on each of these activities. You might do some type of gift giveaway, which is an excellent opportunity to have students provide their names and addresses so that you can begin to develop a mailing list. You could use your list to mail congratulation notes after graduation.

Ambassadors for your facility

The therapists already working at your facility make great ambassadors who can share their knowledge and provide real insight into your facility and working in healthcare.

Encourage your best therapists to give guest lectures at schools. You could offer a mentoring program in which your staff agrees to serve as mentors for students in the final two years of their educational program. Make sure your mentors are great ambassadors for your organization, and that they provide challenging and rewarding student learning experiences.

In students' final semesters, many begin to see how their knowledge and skills actually contribute to positive patient outcomes. This is a real ego booster for them, and they really enjoy the patient and clinical experiences on those units.

Support the schools and students

Offer to help the allied health programs improve student retention, as some programs lose a large percentage of their entering classes. More efficient programs provide more graduates, from which a larger number can be recruited by your organization.

Some schools require therapy volunteer or work assistant experience prior to entering a program to make sure the student understands the realities of working in healthcare. Healthcare organizations can capitalize on this opportunity to provide entry-level jobs and volunteer programs, because it helps you to develop a relationship with the student, provides needed volunteers, and gives the hospital a good look at the student's abilities and work ethic.

Another strategy you might consider is funding scholarships for allied health students and offering loan forgiveness when a student signs on as a new graduate. Scholarships, for example, can have a fixed amount, such as $1,500 per year, or comprise full and partial scholarships. These types of awards often require a payback work commitment per year of funding. They usually focus on junior or senior students. The payoffs for this in therapy assistant programs can be more immediate.

Also consider developing an emergency fund for students in collaboration with local educational programs. Excellent students may be forced to drop out of a program because of small financial needs, such as an unplanned family emergency. Therefore, establish an annual budget—for example, $5,000—and tell faculty to let you know if emergency assistance is needed. Either mail or hand-deliver the check, along with a card that says, "We're investing in you because we think you'll make a great healthcare professional."

Incorporate students into your workplace, and develop stellar mentor programs. Ask for volunteers for the programs, and use only those therapists who demonstrate strong interpersonal skills. Mentors are ambassadors for your facility and can make or break possibilities of a future hire. Hire students as therapy techs, and develop quality internship and externship programs. These programs give students an opportunity to learn about the realities of working with you, and they give you a chance to observe their work ethic and potential. Develop an orientation program, which can be individualized to transition the new grad into the workplace.

Negotiate creative educational programs to increase capacity

Look for opportunities to expand your local healthcare professional programs. Negotiate to offer the following types of programs. Be prepared to provide financial and resource assistance to get these programs up and running.

Multiple graduations

Rather than offering entry in the fall and graduation in the spring, ask programs to consider continuous entry and graduation. Graduations occur in spring, summer, and fall, and you do not have to over-hire in the spring to meet expected vacancies for the year.

Evening and weekend programs

There's a large cohort of second-career individuals who are interested in healthcare but who can't afford to stop work to attend school full time. Evening and weekend programs provide a workable option for those individuals to enter the healthcare work force.

On-site programs

Whether the programs are for therapy tech, therapy assistant, or therapist, providing them on-site makes educational advancement more accessible to your current employees. Provide financial support and flexible scheduling options to encourage participation and success.

Online programs

Negotiate with colleges and universities to offer online academic programs and to help with clinical experiences. Staff members can complete courses from the comfort of their homes. Consider installing a computer lab or developing a computer loan or subsidy program.

Accelerated programs

Accelerated programs meet the needs of second-career individuals who already have a bachelor's degree and are interested in becoming therapists. Programs usually can be completed in a faster time frame.

Educational programs are your best renewable resource for healthcare professionals. Delivery of quality healthcare and services in your community requires close working relationships between education and service-delivery organizations. Analyze your work force needs. Identify the resources each can contribute. Develop creative solutions, and negotiate win-win solutions and educational programs that meet the evolving healthcare and work force needs in your community.

Chapter 10

The power of metrics

The power of metrics in recruitment and retention

More and more healthcare organizations are making work force development and planning an important part of organizational management. Traditionally, some employers have viewed healthcare professionals as readily available commodities that can easily be purchased with sign-on bonuses, higher salaries, benefits, and other incentives as needed. With the current therapy shortage and consumer demands for quality care, employers are moving rapidly to conduct work force and workplace data collection and analysis systematically as an integral component for developing, retaining, and ensuring a high-quality healthcare work force and workplace.

Planning for and ensuring that you have a quality healthcare work force and workplace is a major challenge. Let's consider, for example, that a healthcare organization has 1,200 employees. These employees comprise a wide variety of healthcare professions, managers, and support personnel. Consider the different levels of educational preparation, ages, and cultural backgrounds. Each employee has her or his own thoughts, ideas, and motivators. Each brings different knowledge, skills, and expertise to the workplace. The individual human capital that each contributes can seem abstract until you identify methods for measuring it, and the same holds true for determining costs for turnover and being able to compare your success in recruiting and retaining staff members. Furthermore, consider the millions of processes that occur on a daily basis in an organization that provides healthcare. All of these things can be measured and the results used for planning and improvements.

Making sense of metrics

The goal of metrics is to define it, measure it, and manage it. "It" can be whatever you'd like it to be. Work force metrics are rapidly evolving as an integral component of managing a healthcare organization. The term "metrics" is becoming one of the buzzwords of the 21st century in work force development, and even consumers are beginning to ask, "What do your metrics look like?" Actually, they should be asking, "Which types of metrics are you using?" because there are so many different processes or outcomes you can measure. The possibilities are endless.

What is a metric?

A metric is a measurement of an activity, process, or other function. It involves data collection, analysis, and reporting, usually in a table or graphics format. Sometimes it's simply numbers or a prioritized list. Most often the data are quantitative and numerical in nature. Using metrics allows you to measure your organization's performance and progress over time or make a comparison to another unit, organization, or national or health system norm. Examples of human resource metrics recommended by the American Society of Hospital Human Resources Administrators include:

- Average net revenue per full-time equivalent (FTE)

- Average net operating expense per FTE

- Average compensation expense as a percentage of total operating expense

- Average benefit expense per FTE

- Average recruitment expense per hire

- Vacancy rates

- Retention rates

- Turnover rates

As you can see, many of these metrics specifically demonstrate the overall performance of the organization and the human resources department. You may want to consider factors and measurements that more specifically demonstrate performance of healthcare professionals, such as speech–language pathologists or physical therapists with whom you work—or even the unit you work on, such as the skilled rehab or outpatient clinic. Think critically about the types of data you need for daily decision-making. Effective use of work force data can be a key tool to ensuring a quality staff and workplace.

What do you do with the data?

By analyzing metrics over time, you can establish benchmarks, or standardized measurements (usually averages) that allow you to compare your performance over time or against other units or healthcare organizations. Make sure when you're comparing your metrics to others that data are defined, collected, and analyzed in a similar manner. When comparing metrics, always make sure you are comparing apples to apples, rather than apples to apricots. The first two letters of the words "apples" and "apricots" are the same, but the other letters are very different. The same can hold true for metrics—they can initially appear, sound, and look the same, but they may measure entirely different processes or outcomes.

Some managers use dashboards, which are collections of key performance indicators organized and presented in a format that is easy to read and review. Charts, graphs, and gauges are provided in a consistent format to assist strategic decision-making. Types of data that may be used to form one or more hospital dashboards include:

- Financial and funds management

- Length of stay

- Medication services

- Mortality rates

- Patient demographics

- Patient satisfaction

- Resource management

- Total admissions

- Unplanned returns to surgery

Each metric can help the manager or administrator to determine how the organization performs in the various areas and in what areas changes or corrections may be needed.

Work closely with human resources

Work closely with your human resources department as you consider developing metrics, benchmarks, or dashboards—you might be surprised at the data already being collected in your organization. With the use of computerized systems, much data is readily available. Be sure to collect data on a "need to know" rather than "nice to know" basis, and be very specific about what you need to make work force and workplace decisions.

Traditionally, human resources personnel have provided oversight of salaries and benefits, and other areas such as employee rights. Their roles have recently expanded to encompass strategic planning that includes the development of performance improvement measurements, and other work force metrics and benchmarks. Talk with individuals in your human resources department concerning metrics and benchmarks that will meet your work force planning needs. For instance, you may notice that you have many older therapists in your system and you'd like to determine the proportion that is within five years of the average retirement age.

Principles of human capital metrics

Hold discussions with your fellow managers or with the staff to consider which work force or workplace data you'll want to collect. Consider the following principles.

Never collect data for the sake of collecting data

There's always a cost involved in data collection, whether in time or in other resources. Even the time it takes for you to review the report is an important resource. Therefore, make sure you have a good rationale for how the information will help you in your decision-making process. Consider up-front the amount of time needed to analyze data and turn it into useful information. Never collect data if it will not be analyzed.

Remember to measure processes, not people

Quantifying human capital in your organization is about measuring processes that occur or don't occur within your unit or organization. Consider measuring recruitment, hiring, orientation, learning, and retention processes. The goal is to identify what's working well and what improvements can make it work better.

Keep it flexible: Measure anything you want, in any way you want

When considering a purchase of a traction table, you might be interested in determining the average number of times the piece of technology is actually used in a day to help you decide precisely how many to buy. You can certainly be flexible in how you take your measurements, but be aware that if you plan to observe for trends over time or you would like to compare your findings with other units or organizations, you'll need to define precisely what you're measuring and use the same measurement methods as those with whom you plan to compare your findings.

Measure consistently and use standard formulas

Using a standard formula and similar measurement processes allows you to make comparisons. If you measure your department's vacancies in a unique manner that no one else uses, you cannot compare that figure with other organizations. Determine the type of data measurement you'll use. Most likely it will be quantitative, but you may find at times that qualitative data collection is your most appropriate method. Define your unit of measurement as one or more specific units or an entire organization. For example, is the vacancy rate you're discussing for the physical therapy, occupational therapy, or speech–language pathology department?

Also consider how often you'd like your measurements, such as weekly, monthly, or annually.

Make your metric simple

Don't make your metric more complicated than it has to be. Keep it simple. Define it, explain your measurement method, and be clear about what it does or does not include. For example, a colleague might ask you how many physical therapists work in your inpatient rehab facility. Your first question is to establish whether he or she is interested in staff therapists in a staff physical therapy position, or all physical therapists, since physical therapists work in the roles of supervisor, manager, department head, and so on.

Let's say the colleague wants to measure the number of staff physical therapists, but the assistant rehab manager, who is a physical therapist, spends at least 50% of his or her time providing direct care—should that person be included? You can decide by defining staff physical therapists as those who spend at least 50% of their work time providing direct patient care.

Your next question might be whether he or she wants the total number of staff physical therapists or the number of FTEs. FTEs would be based on the total hours worked, and because you have full-time and part-time positions, that number would be less than your total number of staff physical therapists. It can get pretty complicated. So, if you only need to know the total number of staff physical therapists, keep it simple, and count the number of staff physical therapist names currently with a patient schedule.

Make sure you're measuring what you want to measure

Make sure you're measuring what you actually want to measure. Turnover data is a useful example. You might call it "total turnover" rather than "turnover" if you're interested in the total number of employees who move from one position to another. Both "voluntary turnover" and "involuntary turnover" could comprise "total turnover." Voluntary turnover would include those employees who requested a position change or voluntarily terminated their position. Involuntary turnover includes employees for whom management mandated a position change or terminated their position. You may be interested in breaking your total turnover into "position changes" and "resignations and terminations." You can look at data in several different ways. Just make sure you're measuring what you want to measure.

Measure what's causing you the most pain

How do you know what to measure first? Determine what's causing the biggest issue among your staff. Use feedback from your employee satisfaction surveys, exit interview data, and performance appraisals. Maybe it seems to you that you're losing a large number of therapists on your day shift, or maybe it seems to take forever to get new staff members hired onto your unit. There's a world of things you can measure, but measure what's causing you the most pain and what is most likely to help you make decisions.

Healthcare work force and workplace metrics

As mentioned earlier, you do not need to measure every workplace process. Rather, identify the primary areas where you would like to improve and collect data that you feel will help you in the decision-making process. You may feel external pressure to have some metrics available to show information about your facility. For example, new physical therapy graduates may request to review the following metrics before they accept a position in your healthcare facility:

- PT vacancy rate

- PT turnover rate

- Patient satisfaction scores

- Employee satisfaction scores

- Average tenure of therapy staff, billing staff, front desk staff, etc.

- Education mix of therapy staff

Practical examples of recruitment and retention data you can use to manage your work force

The following are some of the more common findings that are collected in hospitals and healthcare organizations on a regular basis.

Recruitment metrics

A number of measurements may be used to gauge recruitment success:

- **Number of open positions:** This includes the total number of unfilled positions in an organization or on a unit.

- **Days to fill/hire:** This figure defines a day as 24 hours and is calculated from the date you post a position until the date the position is accepted.

- **Days to start:** This finding is computed from the date the position is posted until the date the new hire begins work.

- **Cost per hire:** This figure may only include advertising costs for a position. More recently, organizations are including orientation, decreased productivity, and other costs that are involved with fully incorporating new employees.

- **Number of hires by source:** This usually identifies employees based on where they were prior to the hire. For example, it may be a hospital or it may be an educational program. Be clear about this figure, because it may also refer to how you're reaching your hires by advertising source. Did they learn about your openings by one of your newspaper or journal advertisements?

- **Net gain/loss per month:** This includes the number of hires minus the number that exited your system.

Hiring process metrics

You may be interested in using a variety of metrics to improve your hiring process and even the quality of potential candidates you're attracting:

- **Number of applications:** This is the total number of completed applications you receive. You can tally them by position opening, but most often it is a total of all applications received on a monthly basis.

- **Application/interview ratio:** This is the total number of interviews divided by the total number of completed applications received.

- **Interview/hire ratio:** This is the total number of hires divided by the total number of interviews conducted.

- **Job offer declines by reason:** This is a listing of rationale or comments concerning why a job offer is declined by a candidate.

- **Number of contract staff/contract labor hours:** This is the number of contract staff used on the unit or in the organization and the total number of contract labor hours used.

Orientation process metrics

Organizations are realizing the importance of a quality orientation and quality data, which can help you to rapidly integrate new employees into your work setting:

- **Competencies:** Through either testing or a self-rated competency scale, employers identify skills and competencies of new hires. Competencies are based upon job descriptions and work responsibilities, and learning plans are created to develop individual competency needs.

- **Satisfaction:** This includes feedback from new hires within the first month concerning how satisfied they are with the orientation process and work setting.

- **Length of orientation:** This is the amount of time, usually in months and days, before the employee is able to work independently.

Retention metrics

Measurements pertaining to retention can help you determine areas that need immediate attention, and can help you with your long-term work force planning:

- **Vacancy rate:** Usually vacancy rates include open positions divided by total positions on a unit or in an organization.

- **Turnover rates:** Turnover rates usually include staff departures divided by total positions in a unit or an organization.

- **Percent of new hires:** Percent of new hires is calculated by dividing the total number of new hires by the total number of employees. If you're calculating it for a unit, you use unit hires and unit employees. For the organization, you use total new hires and total employees.

- **Turnover rate of new hires:** This is calculated by dividing the number of new hires who depart by the total number of new hires.

- **Internal promotions:** This includes the number of employees promoted from one role or position to another in your organization.

- **Number of terminations:** This includes the number of employees for whom management or human resources terminates employment.

- **Average length of service:** Dividing the sum of months worked by current employees by the total number of employees will provide the average months of employment of current employees.

- **Percent of employees eligible to retire without penalty:** This is calculated by dividing the number of employees who may retire with no penalty from your pension plan by the total number of employees.

- **Turnover rate of employees eligible to retire without penalty:** This is calculated by dividing the number of employees who actually do retire by the total number of employees.

Whether you're conducting work force planning, improving your recruitment and retention efforts, or building a case for increasing your recruitment and retention budget, metrics are powerful persuaders. Human capital may seem to be a challenge, but metrics provide the hard facts, numbers, and outcomes. Work force data collection, analysis, and review can help you ensure that you have a well-prepared healthcare work force, an exceptional workplace, and quality patient care.

Dos and don'ts of recruitment

Learn from the experiences of others

These top tips of what to do and what not to do will guide you in developing a process for recruiting or help you improve what you are already doing. With more organizations sharing information and networking on issues related to recruiting therapists, it is easy to find out what others are doing that works or doesn't work. Once you identify processes, start developing your own list, and share it with the managers in your organization.

Top 10 things not to do in recruitment

Tip #1: Don't make statements about the work environment that are not true

We all want our workplaces to sound like the place to be, but exaggerating and misrepresenting what you have to offer is inappropriate. Attentive, newly hired therapists are going to realize very quickly that the picture you painted at the interview is not what they are seeing. Therefore, be realistic and honest about your work setting: We all have employees who we wish worked for another department, and many of us hope for the day when we can update the physical layout or appearance of the workplace. Although you don't want to emphasize these points, respond honestly to the questions posed to you at interviews.

Be honest

Prospective employee: "How do people around here get along with each other? At the last place I worked, there was a lot of interdisciplinary tension on our rehab unit."

Manager: "We realize the importance of a professional work environment and never tolerate disruptive behavior in any of our departments. But as you know, there will always be some people with behaviors that may make you uncomfortable. Part of my job, which I take very seriously, is to be responsive to staff members when they identify unacceptable behaviors. I cannot recall any scenarios in which we had severe interdisciplinary issues among our team here, but we have had our disagreements, as everyone does at times."

Tip #2: Don't make promises you cannot keep

Between completing interview sheets, giving tours of the facility, and answering benefit questions, it becomes quite a task to remember all that transpires during the interview process, including what was said. However, the therapists you interview will not forget what you tell them with regard to their schedules, wages, benefits, and so on. If you tell an interviewee, who informs you that he or she has already bought plane tickets, that if he or she is hired you can grant his or her request for the week of Christmas off, you have trapped yourself and the rest of your staff. Therefore, always think the situation through, and imagine various "what if" scenarios. What if one staff member is out on medical leave and another delivers her baby two months early? How are you going to keep your promise for the new hire to still have the holiday off? How will staff members with whom you currently work feel about a new hire getting Christmas off?

Instead of making verbal promises, put in writing anything you do promise, and mail or give the person you interviewed a copy of the document.

Tip #3: Don't allow recruitment to overshadow retention

Recruitment has long been the focus in rehab, particularly considering the state of the current therapy shortage. But increasingly lavish incentives thrown at new therapists can rankle existing employees and make them feel abandoned and ignored. Don't offer incentives and attention to new employees at the expense of those you already have.

Pay attention to your advertising in newspapers and other venues, as not only job seekers will see these ads—your current staff will as well. Therefore, include your retention efforts in those advertisements. Also incorporate an internal advertising campaign to promote retention. Creating a workplace culture that focuses on retention is one of your best recruitment strategies.

Tip #4: Don't allow staff members with unacceptable behavior to continue "bad-mouthing" the department or organization

Set very clear expectations with all staff members regarding this behavior, as it not only damages staff morale, but also diminishes recruitment and retention efforts. Always remember, if they are willing to express negative opinions about the organization at work, just imagine what they are saying in the checkout line at the grocery store. A good place to start working on this issue is with staff members who are in a supervisor-type position. Work with them through role-playing and scripting for appropriate responses that will help to squelch this unacceptable behavior. Encourage the staff to address negative comments on the spot, and direct individuals making the complaints to a forum where their complaints can be addressed, such as at staff meetings.

Tip #5: Don't use a "licensed warm body" as a criterion for meeting recruitment goals

Numerous pressures are placed on recruiters and hiring managers to meet recruitment goals. Some may feel so desperate that they resort to saying, "If they're licensed and breathing, hire them." It's tempting to interview and hire anyone who meets the minimum criteria, particularly for high-demand, revenue-producing positions, but don't fall into that trap. The long-term costs in turnover, team morale, and productivity can be extreme if you hire an individual who doesn't fit. Most employees will tell you they would rather work short-staffed than bring the wrong team member on board.

One strategy to consider is to use temporary staff until you find the right professional for your unit. Reassure recruiters, managers, and the staff that although it is important to get the position filled, it is critical that you fill it with a person who can contribute significantly to your organizational goal of quality patient care.

Tip #6: Don't dwell on your or your organization's limitations

Some organizations seem to have all the bells and whistles when it comes to recruiting, and the grass often looks greener in a competing facility. But be sure to focus on your organization's strengths. What keeps you there? Ask new and seasoned staff members the same question. Talk these points up with potential candidates. Identify organizational limitations, and develop strategies for improvement.

Tip #7: Don't neglect recruitment infrastructure

It's amazing how many people think recruiters live glamorous lives, and how exciting it must be to travel and talk with people. But in reality, many functions and responsibilities are included in the role, and it can be lonely and challenging to fulfill them, especially if you're the only one in your organization doing it.

Set a long-term goal to develop a recruitment army. Equip employees in your organization to share the benefits of working there, and work with your staff development department to design a "My Stories" seminar. Encourage each employee in your organization to participate and to develop personal stories about how they make a difference in your organization. Discuss forums where these could be shared in public, such as at cookouts, at community gatherings, and through letters to the editor of your local newspaper. Hold a follow-up group session to discuss responses.

Establish a community healthcare roundtable to discuss healthcare personnel recruitment issues. Conduct regional work force analysis to identify high-priority personnel needs. If you know physical therapy will be a long-term need, work with physical therapy training programs to increase enrollment and graduations. Work together to develop creative work force development programs, and apply collectively for funding from the U.S. Department of Labor, the U.S. Health Resources and Services Administration, or even private philanthropies that focus on healthcare access.

Tip #8: Don't expect sign-on incentives to retain staff members

Sign-on bonuses can get an active or passive job seeker's attention, but most likely they will not be the sole reason an individual will agree to work with you. They can help motivate new hires to stay for the length of the sign-on agreement, but you must have a great work culture to retain them for the long term.

Tip #9: Don't allow rehab areas to operate revolving recruitment doors

Maintain turnover data on a departmental basis. Identify those that have high turnover rates and determine what's causing the turnover. Analyze employee satisfaction and exit interview data, and compare and contrast findings among the different units. Meet with the unit manager and employees to discuss the data, and identify issues that might influence employee retention. Develop an action plan. Identify a responsible and accountable employee or committee to develop a timeline and oversee its implementation.

Tip #10: Don't spend time on strategies that aren't producing recruits

Analyze your recruitment strategies to determine which are producing results and which are not. You can add codes to the advertisements you place in a variety of media so that you can determine how candidates learned about your openings. When potential candidates contact your recruitment office, ask them to describe where they saw the advertisement or provide you with the advertisement code. When you exhibit at career fairs, get an estimate of the number of people who attend the fair, the number who stop by your booth, the number who leave names and addresses, and the number who actually interview with you. If strategies are not producing desired results, consider setting them aside. Of course, one of your aims is to promote a positive image and create good will, so not all strategies will produce concrete results. But your time is valuable, and you want to make sure your total efforts produce recruitment results.

Top 10 things to do in recruitment

Tip #1: Do improve your interviewing skills

How you present yourself and the questions you pose during the interview process affect the perceptions of the prospective hire. Be prepared for the interview by having your desk presentable, having important documents on hand (such as the job description), and ensuring uninterrupted time, when possible. Seek input from staff members regarding questions they would like to see included during the interview. Don't discount the idea of also having staff members interview the candidate—after all, they are the ones who will be working side by side with the new therapist. The interview process should not be one-sided, so provide candidates with time to conduct their own interviews of you and the department.

Tip #2: Do involve the staff in all recruitment processes

Giving staff members the opportunity to be involved in the interview process is just one method of getting them involved in recruitment. Ask the staff to preview advertisements before they go to print to offer a reality check, and make sure you are not promoting a process that doesn't actually take place in the department. Encourage staff members to accompany the recruiter to recruitment fairs or to meet with high school seniors on career day.

Make time to educate staff members on the correct response to the questions that are most commonly posed to the recruiter. Your staff members will be unable to do their part in recruitment if they are not well versed on matters such as employee benefits and new community services. Share with them what types of social situations are great opportunities for recruitment, such as when they hear about a new coworker at a family member's job whose spouse "happens to be a therapist."

Tip #3: Do identify and know your competition

Conduct a competition analysis to identify organizations you compete with for different types of personnel. Compare and contrast work cultures, opportunities for advancement, and types of units, specialties, and programs. Know the strengths of your organization, and be enthusiastic about sharing information on your outstanding programs and retention rates. Never make negative statements or comments about your competition; instead, redirect the conversation to discuss more positive aspects of your organization.

Tip #4: Do optimize Internet and e-recruitment technologies

Organizations are recruiting large proportions of healthcare professionals through use of the Internet. Make sure your "Job opportunities" button is on your organization's home page and that it links directly to up-to-date, user-friendly job listings. Allow for immediate submission of applications and resumes online, and offer to answer questions by e-mail or by phone. Most hospital and healthcare Web sites are designed to attract patients, so review your site to make sure it also provides positive images that attract potential candidates. Stay away from spam recruitment messages, but certainly consider low-cost e-cards as an alternative to direct-mail campaigns. Look for strategies to keep you informed on the latest electronic recruiting technologies, and for major initiatives, consider outsourcing to high-tech recruitment agencies.

Tip #5: Do publicly brag about your outstanding staff members in newspaper articles, journals, and other venues

Job-hunting professionals want to know about staff members with whom they may work. When they read about staff members who have attained certifications or volunteered for a community effort, they receive a message that the organization supports professional development. The more they see these public declarations of accomplishments, the stronger their perception that your organization supports its therapists and offers many opportunities. It also directly affects retention, as staff members love the accolades they receive when people they know see a photo or advertisement in the paper about their new certification. When announcing major physical changes to the organization, include photos of staff members along with pictures of the upgraded facility.

Tip #6: Do embrace opportunities to work with schools of physical therapy, occupational therapy, and speech–language pathology

Due to the shortage of faculty at many professional therapy training schools, many are having trouble meeting their classroom goals, as well as those for the clinical setting. Collaborate with the training schools, and create a wonderful opportunity to showcase student therapists all you have to offer in your facility. During their clinical rotations, students will be working alongside your staff and will be able to picture themselves there as a staff member. During their time on duty, existing staff members will be able to get a feel for the characters and personalities of the prospective hires. Should they decide to apply for a position with you when they graduate, you will already have an idea whether you want them as part of the team. Remember, skills can often be taught later on, but character and passion for a career in patient care must be there from the beginning.

Tip #7: Do set a personal goal to develop every inquiry into a job application

When you make the first contact with a prospective hire—whether via a face-to-face meeting at a career fair exhibit or an e-mail or phone inquiry—set a personal goal that this individual will visit your office for an interview. Of course, he or she must meet the job requirements for the position, but with recruiting experience and expertise, you often can determine within the first few moments whether the candidate is a good fit for your organization. Keep your own tally of how many got away and how many were hired.

Tip #8: Do market your organization in a thousand places rather than one

It's wise to remember the old saying, "Don't put all your eggs in one basket," when considering marketing your organization. That is, don't invest your entire advertising budget in one resource, such as a newspaper or journal. Rather, use several media outlets to increase your individual and target group reach. Use a variety of media and face-to-face strategies to get the word out about how great it is to work with your organization. Consider marketing strategies such as trumpeting your Magnet designation or any national unit and specialty recognition awards. These types of outside recognition validate quality care and excellent workplaces.

Tip #9: Do establish trusting relationships

Honesty and integrity are two of the most important qualities of a great recruiter. Relationships with recruits begin at your first point of contact. Although it may be difficult to do on a day-to-day basis, make sure you are attentive and fully engaged in the moment. Listen to their interests and concerns. Keep hiring managers informed of prospects, and provide consistent follow-up. Be professional and collegial with peer recruiters. If a prospect's background and skills are a better fit for a competing organization in your region, make the referral by giving your peer recruiter a call. Think about it: The prospect was not a good fit for your organization, but if he or she is a good fit for the other facility, you suddenly have two individuals at your competitor's organization singing your organization's praises.

Tip #10: Do spend time with colleagues who mentor, coach, and suggest ways to improve your recruitment skills

Everyone must seek ways to improve, and mentors are a wonderful way to fast-track your learning and development. Identify areas you would like to improve, and then consider leaders who can help develop this expertise, which may come in the form of knowledge or via professional contacts. Be aware that the mentors who may help you most may be outside of your normal practice arena. Spend time with people who build you up, rather than tear you down.

Chapter 12

What's working in the non-healthcare environment?

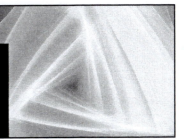

Differentiate yourself from your competitors

Healthcare is a world of rules, regulations, and requirements specific to our service. We tend to stay within our own group when looking for resources, answers, and ideas on how to improve what we do. Managers participate in seminars geared only for the world of healthcare, and the journals they read are directed at the same audience. Sometimes we forget there is another world out there dealing with the same management challenges we have, including recruitment and retention.

For example, it is not easy to recruit and retain people to work at a fast-food restaurant chain when there are six more companies just like them on the same street. These companies address the same questions of how to compete when everyone pays the same starting wage. Or they put money and time into orienting new people, just as in healthcare, only to find employees lured away to a place that will pay them more. Other industries also face the challenge of meeting difficult scheduling needs. For example, would you want to be working by yourself at a convenience store on the midnight shift and have to close out the cash register? We have more in common with other industries than most of us realize, and it's time to look at how the other side of the business world confronts some of these challenges successfully.

Surprising the customer

Many leadership lessons can be learned from observing what non-healthcare organizations do to encourage their employees and many of these successful principles could be applied to healthcare.

Checking in

I was checking in at the front desk of a hotel, when suddenly the young woman who was helping me stepped out from behind the counter. I thought she was heading that way to do something else, and I was taken aback when I realized she was simply coming around to talk to me. She handed me my room key and discussed local information. When I asked her why she stepped out from behind the counter, she explained that her company's goal is to make the customer feel special and like an individual, and they realized that talking to the customer from behind a desk is very impersonal. I was very impressed by this attitude, but I wondered how the employees felt about doing it. The young woman replied that she thought it was a great idea, as she had never liked having a counter between her and the people she was helping. The hotel kept me as a customer, even though they charged more per night than many others.

Customer service

You can see parallels between this behavior and those in your own workplace. Imagine if one of your employees approached the receptionist in personnel with a question about his paycheck. The receptionist is on the phone when the therapist approaches, and it is obvious that she is on a personal call. How important would you feel to the organization if you were this therapist taking time from your break to do this? Compare that to the receptionist who concludes the call quickly and makes immediate eye contact with that therapist. It sends a message that the employee is important and has your attention right now.

Shared goals

I arrived at a supply store a few minutes before they were due to open. It was a nice day, so I decided to wait outside for the short period of time. Looking into the front window, I noticed that all the employees gathered around one person for what looked like a meeting. When it was over, just before they unlocked the doors, I noticed all the staff members got together and applauded. After completing my shopping, I asked the man at the checkout about what I had witnessed through the window. He informed me that it was their daily "pep" talk with their manager and that the applause was them congratulating one another for meeting a team goal that they had set.

Teams are made up of individuals

Making staff members feel like they're part of a team is a crucial element for retention, but if no one recognizes what people bring to the table as individuals, where is the motivation to hang around with the organization? At the weekly staff meeting in your department, make time to recognize what the group and individuals have accomplished. The supervisor or manager does this in your absence, not necessarily every day, but on a regular basis to encourage and motivate the staff.

Keeping up with the changing workplace

A healthcare manager's greatest challenge continues to be difficulty in changing with the times and moving past old habits of management. Keeping up with the changing work force is essential to successful businesses and has allowed them not only to attract the best employees, but also to keep them around. Concepts that appeal to the changing work force include telecommuting, job-sharing, and flexible work hours and days.

Value employees as people

In this day and age of iPods, podcasts, and YouTube, we find ourselves moving away from pen and paper. Although e-mail communication or a text message is effective, sometimes a handwritten note can accomplish much more: It sends a message that you took the extra time to hand-write a message of importance.

An electronic instrument manufacturer started a "You Done Good Award," which is simply a printed note card that employees can send to one another. The cards have become important enough to the organization and the people who work there that those who receive one display it proudly on their desk. The communications manager for this company noted that even when people say nice things to you, it means more when people take the time to write their name on a piece of paper to say it.[1]

Recognition

In some car-manufacturing companies, employees involved in the manufacturing process get to actually sign their name on some part of the product. It is a representation of their involvement in developing this product.

As another example, you can walk onto a Southwest Airlines aircraft and see a plaque in the cabin that recognizes an employee for his or her service loyalty. In each monthly issue of the airline's magazine, there is a story with a photo about one of the employees and how he or she has contributed to the company's success. Whether it is autographing a product or putting the employee's photo in a magazine, the recognition is clear to everyone, especially that employee.

Spirit of fun

Some industries have discovered the value of making the workplace fun. Southwest Airlines' employees work hard, but they have fun at the same time. The company encourages committees that arrange fun employee activities, and although they are in a very serious business, staff members know that acceptable humor at the right time is supported and encouraged from the top.

Other examples of ways employers have incorporated fun into the workplace include the following:

- A small, privately owned manufacturing company produces products that require extreme concentration at the individual workstations. Unannounced, the manager showed up with several rented vans and shut down the shop for part of the day. He took everyone out for ice cream and then to an arcade, where he handed each person tokens to play the games.

- A group of government employees had been working hard toward meeting a team goal that they eventually achieved. One afternoon, they were called into the manager's office and were handed movie tickets for that afternoon's show. The spontaneous act made the employees feel like kids playing hooky from school and allowed them to have fun as a group.[2]

- A kitchen appliance assembly plant is located in the stifling South of the country. Despite the presence of fans, during the summer it is a challenge for the employees to stay motivated and meet production expectations. One day, employees see one of the managers walking through the plant handing out popsicles—simple yet important to the staff.

These examples may seem impossible to duplicate in healthcare—you can't shut down a therapy department in order to take people to a bowling alley. But it's important to note that it is not so much what you do as how unexpected the action is.

When you read the business section of the newspaper, start to look for stories about what other businesses are doing to recognize, recruit, and retain employees. Although you may not be able to do exactly the same things they are doing, their actions should help you come up with some great ideas of your own. How about initiating an employee support account for each department's budget that gives the manager funds throughout the year to purchase items such as movie tickets, ice cream, pizza deliveries, or pens? Surprise the staff with the unexpected, and the return on your investment will show up in your retention statistics.

Use your Web site

A quick Internet search of many well-known corporations with reputations for success in the area of recruitment and retention reveals one important fact: The companies have pages on their Web sites dedicated to the individual and team achievements of their employees. Some have employee photos, quotes, information on the charities the employees select to sponsor, photos of company events, and so on.

Most health organizations have Web sites, and it is time to take advantage of the power of the Internet. Use this opportunity to show employees that they are so integral to the operation of the hospital that you are posting employee photos, accomplishments, and achievements right on the Web site. People love to go online or call their families and friends to tell them to look on the hospital Web site for their picture or story.

Best places to work

Business magazines publish lists each year of the "best places to work" in America. The magazines use specific criteria such as benefits, wages, and work flexibility in the selection process. Fortune magazine announced its 2005 winner—Wegmans, a grocery store chain based in Rochester, NY—and stated, "Wegmans does things differently, including the way it deals with employees."[3]

The Wegmans Web site offers 16 good reasons to work there, which range from friendly teams to adoption assistance. It also states: "In order to attract and retain the best people, we offer competitive benefits that make the perfect garnish to the employment experience."[4]

Pizza Hut was voted the best place to work in Dallas by Dallas/Ft Worth Magazine, and the company proudly proclaims, "The only thing that tops our pizza is our people!" The company believes in providing an environment that nurtures staff members and makes them feel that they have contributed to the process. The eight leadership principles the company follows include encouraging everyone to contribute their ideas and state, "We hate bureaucracy and all the nonsense that comes with it."[5]

Auto rental company Avis uses the motto, "We try harder." Of its employees, 18,000 enjoyed the opportunity to be entered into a program that recognized the top 40 examples of employees who had tried harder. Prizes were awarded and their stories posted on the company's Web site.

How the employee perceives he or she is being treated and how you actually treat the employee may be worlds apart, and it is vital that organizations explore this difference. "If you want the customer to be treated like a king, then you have to treat the people you manage like royalty."[6] In Bill Fromm's book, *The 10 Commandments of Business and How to Break Them*, he reflects on a client he had who was rude to his employees to the point of using profanities. Some employees hated coming to work if they knew they were going to have to deal with this client. As the well-being of his people was Fromm's biggest priority, he "fired" the client. Fromm gathered his employees at a meeting, where he announced that he had terminated the relationship with the client. He was received with screams of surprise and applause by his employees, who felt supported by their boss.

Once again, it may seem impossible to relate these examples to your workplace, but with patience and input from the staff, you will be amazed at the difference you can make. Managers need to step up and support and protect those who do their job every day.

Sometimes the customer isn't right

One of my therapists in the outpatient clinic reported a verbally abusive patient with a family member who also made statements that the therapist perceived as threatening. The clinic supervisor was unsuccessful in stemming the abusive situation. The rehab manager called the referring physician to explain the situation and stated that the patient was going to be discharged in order to protect the safety and security of the staff. It's never nice to "fire a patient," but it is important to stand up for employees and protect their safety.

Strategies to make new employees feel welcome

Have you ever considered how much it costs your organization in time and money to orient one new therapist? Many businesses have put a price on orientation and initial training and have related these costs to a sum that equals what they put into recruitment and retention efforts. Would doing anything less make good business sense? Once you have them and they want the job, how important do you make them feel once they are on board? How would you like to start your first day as a new manager with not even a pad of paper on the desk? Remember, you need to put the same efforts for recruitment and retention into the new manager you hire as you do for the staff therapist.

We can learn techniques from the business world to improve our welcome to new therapy managers:

- Have business cards made and ready to go on the first day

- Have the office stocked with office supplies, such as pens, a stapler, and paper

- Place on the new therapy manager's desk an updated company directory of phone numbers and e-mail addresses, his or her pager/cell phone with instructions and numbers, and a welcome note from the organization with a jar of candy

- Arrange for another manager to show up at lunchtime to take the new employee to lunch

- Be sure the new therapy manager's computer is in working order and that any information of a personal nature is removed

- Arrange a manager's breakfast or lunch meeting to introduce the new manager to his or her peer group

- If new managers relocate from another part of the country, mail them packets of information about the community from the Chamber of Commerce, provide them with contact information for reliable realtors, and inquire as to whether they need information about the local schools, places of worship, and other community information

Other techniques employed by businesses to make a good first impression include the following:

- Intel Corporation sends its new hires a packet of material in the mail before they begin employment that reads "Welcome to the World of Intel."

- Gift baskets are sent to the homes of new hires for Quick Solutions.

- An e-mail is sent to all employees of Persistence Software informing them that today a new employee is starting. The company encourages existing staff members to stop by to introduce themselves by placing a tray of breakfast food near the new hire's desk.[7]

All the ideas and creativity you read about should lead you to this one thought: Your ability to show employees that you care about them is an important advantage when faced with the challenges of holding on to good staff members and recruiting the best out there looking for jobs. Regardless of what it costs you in time and money, the effectiveness and success of your actions will be in the emotion of the employees. If they feel like you care about them being a part of your team, you have made an emotional connection with them and will find that they will be committed members of the organization.

References

1. Bob Nelson, *1001 Ways to Reward Employees* (New York: Workman Publishing, 1994): p. 4.

2. Beverly L. Kaye and Sharon Jordan-Evans, *Love 'Em or Lose 'Em: Getting Good People to Stay* (San Francisco: Berrett-Koehler Publishers, 1999): p. 90.

3. Matthew Boyle, "The Wegman Way," Fortune, *http://money.cnn.com/magazines/fortune/fortune_archive/2005/01/24/8234048/index.htm* (accessed August 22, 2007).

4. Wegmans Web site, *www.wegmans.com/about/jobs/benefits.asp* (accessed August 22, 2007).

5. Pizza Hut Web site, *http://www.pizzahut.com/Careers.aspx* (accessed August 22, 2007).

6. Bill Fromm, *The 10 Commandments of Business and How to Break Them* (New York: Berkley Books, 1991).

7. Leigh Branham, *Keeping the People Who Keep You In Business* (New York: AMACOM, 2001).

Additional resources and reference tools

- Timothy Butler, et al., "Job Sculpting: The Art of Retaining Your Best People," *Harvard Business Review* (September–October 1999).

- Robert E. Farrell, *Give 'Em the Pickle* (Portland, OR: Farrell's Pickle Production, Inc., 1995).

- Adrian Gostick, et al., *Managing with Carrots* (Salt Lake City: Gibbs-Smith Publisher, 2001).

- Bob Nelson, *1001 Ways to Energize Employees* (New York: Workman Publishing, 1994).

- Web resources:

  - *www.humanresources.about.com:* extensive resource for all matters related to managing

  - *www.shiftwork.com:* resources for staff members who work the night shift

  - *www.followyourdreams.com:* daily motivational statements and quotes

  - *www.hru.net:* monthly manager tip

  - *www.managementfirst.com:* HR articles, tips, and so on

  - *www.growtalent.com:* survey results on best places to work

  - *www.fastcompany.com:* resource for innovative business practices